Is Your Horse
100%?

Is Your Horse
100%?

**Resolve Painful Limitations in
the Equine Body with Conformation
Balancing and Fascia Fitness**

Margret Henkels

Photographs by Patti Bose • Foreword by Gene Doyle, BCSI

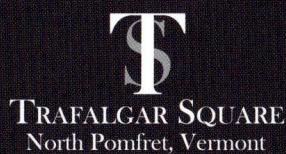

TRAFALGAR SQUARE
North Pomfret, Vermont

First published in 2017 by
Trafalgar Square Books
North Pomfret, Vermont 05053

Disclaimer of Liability
The author and publisher shall have neither liability nor responsibility to any person or entity with respect to any loss or damage caused or alleged to be caused directly or indirectly by the information contained in this book. While the book is as accurate as the author can make it, there may be errors, omissions, and inaccuracies.

Trafalgar Square Books encourages the use of approved safety helmets in all equestrian sports and activities.

Library of Congress Cataloging-in-Publication Data
Names: Henkels, Margret, 1952- author.
Title: Is your horse 100%? : resolve painful limitations in the equine body
   with conformation balancing and fascia fitness / Margret Henkels.
Other titles: Is your horse one hundred percent?
Description: North Pomfret, Vermont : Trafalgar Square Books, 2017. |
   Includes bibliographical references and index.
Identifiers: LCCN 2016044460 | ISBN 9781570767913
Subjects: LCSH: Horses--Conformation. | Horses--Anatomy.
Classification: LCC SF279 .H465 2017 | DDC 636.1--dc23 LC record available at
   https://lccn.loc.gov/2016044460

Photographs by Patti Bose
Book design by Lauryl Eddlemon
Cover design by RM Didier
Index by Andrea M. Jones (www.jonesliteraryservices.com)
Typeface: Open Sans

Printed in China

10 9 8 7 6 5 4 3 2 1

This book is dedicated to horses,
and their people, everywhere.

Contents

PART I

Contents (continued)

PART II

Conformation Balancing: The Fascia-Change Work 47

Contents (continued)

Foreword

In this impressive and important new work Margret Henkels has managed to do the nearly impossible: discuss in clear and concise language subtle expressions of equine pain and discontent through observation of movement loss within the fascial planes. Relevant terms such as *fascial aggregations*, *"stuck" movement patterns*, *correctable abbreviated gait*, and *tail movement assessment* all require a lot of explanation to prepare an individual to correctly look for them, and then be able to see and assess them accurately. Henkels' ability to convey the unspoken language and unseen needs of these wonderful animals—our horses—is truly a part of her gift for working with them as intimately as she does. Her sensitivity and understanding challenge us all to be as apt as she is. Having been lucky enough to see her at work, and doubly lucky to have a trained eye, I can tell you the results—in terms of ease and softness in the resulting animal—were a true joy to observe. It always looks like the subject is going to fall asleep under her hands!

Beginning to discuss fascia entails educating the equestrian population in the newly appreciated and least known physical system of the body. Right along with the digestive, muscular, nervous, and all the other recognized body systems, the fascial system is today being more fully seen and understood for its importance.

For instance, every part of a horse's body is wrapped in fascial "bags"—every bone, every nerve, every muscle. The bags surrounding the muscles lengthen and thicken to create the tendons, and the thick fascial bands surrounding every single joint are known as ligaments. 90 percent of the brain is known to be fascia! All those bags can stick to each other. This stickiness is useful to the body, in support of body shape especially. However, this same quality of stickiness can also work against free and natural movement in the horse's stance and gait, resulting in an undesirable conformation and limited movement possibilities.

Now I'm sure you can more completely understand the timeliness and necessity of the beauty and economy offered by Margret Henkels' Conformation Balancing system. Full movement efficiency and ease in your mount can only be arrived at after unwanted fascial aggregations are released. In terms of your riding, this work enables the horse to respond more fully to your most subtle commands due to increased calmness and focus.

So welcome to a wonderful new world of awareness around your horse's comfort, your riding goals, and ultimately how you relate to your horse. As a human fascial release practitioner, I can tell you that we two-leggeds always benefit from tissue release, as well, and I have never seen *anyone* who failed to be happier, more pain-free, relaxed, and confident after receiving the work.

We humans have voices to give our approval and thanks for such relief. Try this work, then watch and see how your horse gives his...without saying a word.

Gene Doyle, BCSI
Certified KMI Structural Integration Practitioner

Acknowledgments

It takes a team to produce a book. I am grateful for the talented help and support I received in completing this project, and thanks go to:

The Rancho Mariposa community, especially the horses: Beau, CT, EZ, Jet, Samson, Scout and Remy.

Kleka, my own horse, guided me.

A huge thank you goes to Barbara Brockman, whose support helped the project flow smoothly.

Gratitude goes to Patti Bose, photographer, whose creative talent and love of horses let their spirits shine through in these pictures.

Thanks also to Charles Kacin, artist, whose creative illustrations clarify the vision.

I thank friends and family who supported the path of this book, especially Dr. Robert Schweitzer, DVM, and all my clients and their horses—without them this would be impossible.

Finally, I'm grateful to the Trafalgar Square Books publishing team who supported this process and agreed to bring this book to the equestrian world.

Using This Book

With this book, you'll use my method of Conformation Balancing to successfully bring the horse to 100-percent ability. It's best to read the chapters in order and use the methods as presented.

Part I is an introduction to fascia (connective tissue) and how it structures conformation. It also includes information about how to do a conformation assessment of the horse before starting the Conformation Balancing fascia-change work in Part II. The connection between fascia and conformation is a new concept for many riders, yet fascia controls how the horse looks and moves.

The chapters in Part II show how to work directly on many different parts of the horse's body using various methods of hand contact that promote what I call fascia changes (see p. 12 where I define this). This part also identifies common problems and their solutions, includes specific injury problem-solving suggestions for how to safely return a horse to work after injury or inactivity, as well as offering specific exercises for maintaining range of motion. Finally, I offer a holistic approach to maintaining a horse's fitness through conscious communication with him regarding riding goals. In more detail:

- Chapter 1 describes fascia and how it connects everything in the body, including the emotional aspects of injury.

- Chapter 2 discusses conformation, how to assess it, and record a conformation inventory of your horse.

- A "balanced stance" is the focus of chapter 3, along with safety in horse bodywork as preparation for "investigating" your horse.

- In Part II, chapter 4, I explain how to scan the horse with your hands in order to familiarize yourself with his unique body and condition. Then I discuss the different methods of hand contact used, plus information about the specific areas of the horse's body that you need to balance, including the horse's tail.

- Chapter 5 teaches the three very important areas for work on nearly every horse.

- Solutions for common problems are in chapter 6.

- In chapter 7, you learn to notice the horse's progress and how to help him stabilize the changes with his exercise work.

- Criticism and haste can bring setbacks, so chapter 8 offers help in preventing a slip back into old habits.

- If you'd like a deeper intimacy with your horse, chapter 9 is all about telepathy with horses.

- Chapter 10 shows you a body map for keeping track of your work, the horse's changes, and your new relationship with him.

All along the way, you are following the photo examples for practicing them on your horse to make progress with fitness, even if he lacks obvious major injury or strain.

Don't be concerned if you come to this work fresh, without bodywork experience. Conformation Balancing of fascia is a simple skill somewhat similar to computer work. Just as you develop a "keyboard ability" when you use your computer, your hands learn "kinesthetic ability" when you feel the horse's fascia through his outer skin. I use everyday language, and for simplicity, I have omitted technical terms and descriptions. However, for unusual terms I have included a glossary on page 12.

This book is designed for practical use in the barn or field. Diagnostics and problems more appropriate to veterinary solutions, chiropractic methods, and acupuncture are not included here.

Fascia is a universe of its own. The examples encourage you to use the methods with your horse. This is effective work using sensitivity, good judgment, and, of course, the horse's agreement. Horses do indeed transform with Conformation Balancing. They often become the sport partners we dream of them being, as their old "baggage" and limits dissolve.

Introduction to Conformation Balancing

Clients often ask me how I got into horse myofascial bodywork. A passion for horses, and my own personal experience of being completely healed, brought me to this work—Conformation Balancing. A riding fall at 28 brought chronic injuries lasting years. I knew nothing about fascia (connective tissue) and its role in organizing the entire body. A synchronicity at a horse show introduced me to Steve Evans, a Heller Work practitioner. Heller Work is an offshoot of Rolfing and trains people in its particular approach to fascia. The weekly myofascial-release sessions transformed me into fitness. Each week, for 15 weeks, I drove to Taos where Steve lived and returned feeling better. I loved the changes I felt and the work itself. My experience is that Heller Work is much less strenuous tissue work and is comfortable for the patient, even in the first session, unlike Rolfing, which is known to be strenuous.

On his table, I talked about my horses often and told him stories of my rides. Steve suggested I consider getting into the horse bodywork field. "Just what I need, another startup," I said with a laugh. His suggestion seed grew. The changes I felt transformed my goals. Paperwork and financial data of the business world lost their charm. I felt amazingly better and fit enough to work with horses. He referred me to Equine Natural Movement, Heller for Horses, in Battle Ground, Washington, where I took a module of training, before certifying.

In myofascial-release training, I heard the call of the physical world. And, I learned something completely new: how hidden feelings surface when myofascial cells open as they release compression, and in the process, release trauma that has been held in the body. The emotional and spiritual transformations that occurred during myofascial change fascinated me: this clearing of trauma by bodywork is part of the amazing miracle of myofascial change. In sessions with horses, I watched horses change emotionally and trust me. Horses in pain wanted help. There are many myofascial-modality resources for humans. The work in this book is for the horse.

As it turned out, I focused on solving long-term problems for horses. Horses with elusive, painful disabilities arrived to advance my experience. These talented horses with difficult imbalances challenged me in each session as the horses and I explored their blockages to fitness. Since I knew it was possible to regain 100 percent fitness, I communicated this understanding to them. An anxious horse is a fearful horse, and if we take no notice of his anxiety, or call it laziness or a bad

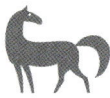

attitude, a horse acts out to save his life, and the dance of dangerous dysfunction begins for the rider—or anyone else working with the horse.

I became very interested in why so many horses didn't look fit. Patterns revealing how these horses became limited and miserable emerged. Digital photos became part of my work and I designed body maps to record the progress. I enjoyed the transformation these horses showed as they returned to fitness and productive lives. The riders were delighted.

Since efficiency in this process is vital, I studied the patterns and the appearances of the horses. Over time, the body limits matched up with certain physical looks, despite the breed, age, or work. Conformation Balancing developed from this process of looking at the horse's conformation and finding his imbalances. It was a major discovery to realize how little genetics or perfect situations could prevent a horse's decline when he had a strain and an accident. The horses were well bred and well trained, but their conformation was unbalanced. The decline in these injured horses mystified their rider. The painful "soft-tissue" problem forces many well-trained and talented horses into a state of idleness, a great loss for both horse and rider.

Like humans, horses are joyful when expressing their gifts and talent. Horses need help for loss of fitness, including their lost happiness as horses, for when a horse isn't fit, he's caught in a primal, cellular panic, fearful that a predator will get him. A numbed state of resistant fear is *not* a happy life for a horse.

> In the Still Point, the horse focuses consciously on his fascia changes, he feels them helping him, while not quite knowing what they are or where they are.

Conformation Balancing was developed to offer tools that any motivated rider can learn to end this cycle of limitation and eruptions of fear by the horse. Our lives as riders depend upon our horses' mental balance and cooperation. Conformation Balancing emphasizes the "Still Point" change for this reason: the Still Point occurs when the horse turns his attention inward as we work with his body to follow his body's myofascial changes. His eye looks very focused and intense as he feels change happening in his tissue. These Still Point changes bring emotional and physical relief. He feels the change and recognizes it as an improvement. These cellular changes are unique to the myofascial-change process.

As riders know well, the horse's emotional experience often rules the day; the importance of the change for the horse in a Still Point is beyond words. Best of all, the myofascial-release methods bring effective, lasting progress and relief.

As with humans, this relief from pain lifts the horse's spirits. The inner change of emotional, physical, and spiritual progress brings him into a new fitness. Since we are offering him relief, a new trust grows. I truly believe that we are on a threshold of change now for horses and humans. The horse's desire is slowly being included in our plans, which is a welcome move forward in the horse/human relationship.

As you'll learn in this book, the head and the tail are the two balance points holding the "internet" or network of the horse's fascia. The head changes offered are essential since horses continually wear bits and halters. We can only dimly imagine the head imbalances that the average horse lives with daily. The tail is a key to hindquarter flexion. Conformation Balancing shows how the simple release of holding the tail in both hands brings miracles to the horse's comfort level.

Fortunately, the resources for myofascial release (commonly called MFR) are expanding rapidly. The book and DVD, *Architecture of Human Living Fascia: Cells and Extracellular Matrix as Revealed by Endoscopy,* by Jean-Claude Guimberteau, MD, opens the world of fascia for a wide audience. Endoscopy reveals the life of fascia cells and the entire extra-cellular matrix. Dr. Guimberteau's fiber-optic surgical equipment shows the visual miracle of fascia. The myofascial release practitioners and teachers trained by John Barnes and Ida Rolf help human clients. John Barnes actively teaches throughout the world. The work of Ida Rolf is continued via her training programs. There are also many other branches of myofascial-release work to research and choose, thanks to the internet.

It is a privilege to work with horses and their human partners as they find enhanced happiness and well-being together. We have much to give back to the horse. Your journey in the horse's fascial "internet" universe will reward you beyond your expectations.

Like electricity, we don't need
to understand fascia to know
it is the connecting tissue that
organizes the entire body.

Conformation Balancing:
Preparatory Work

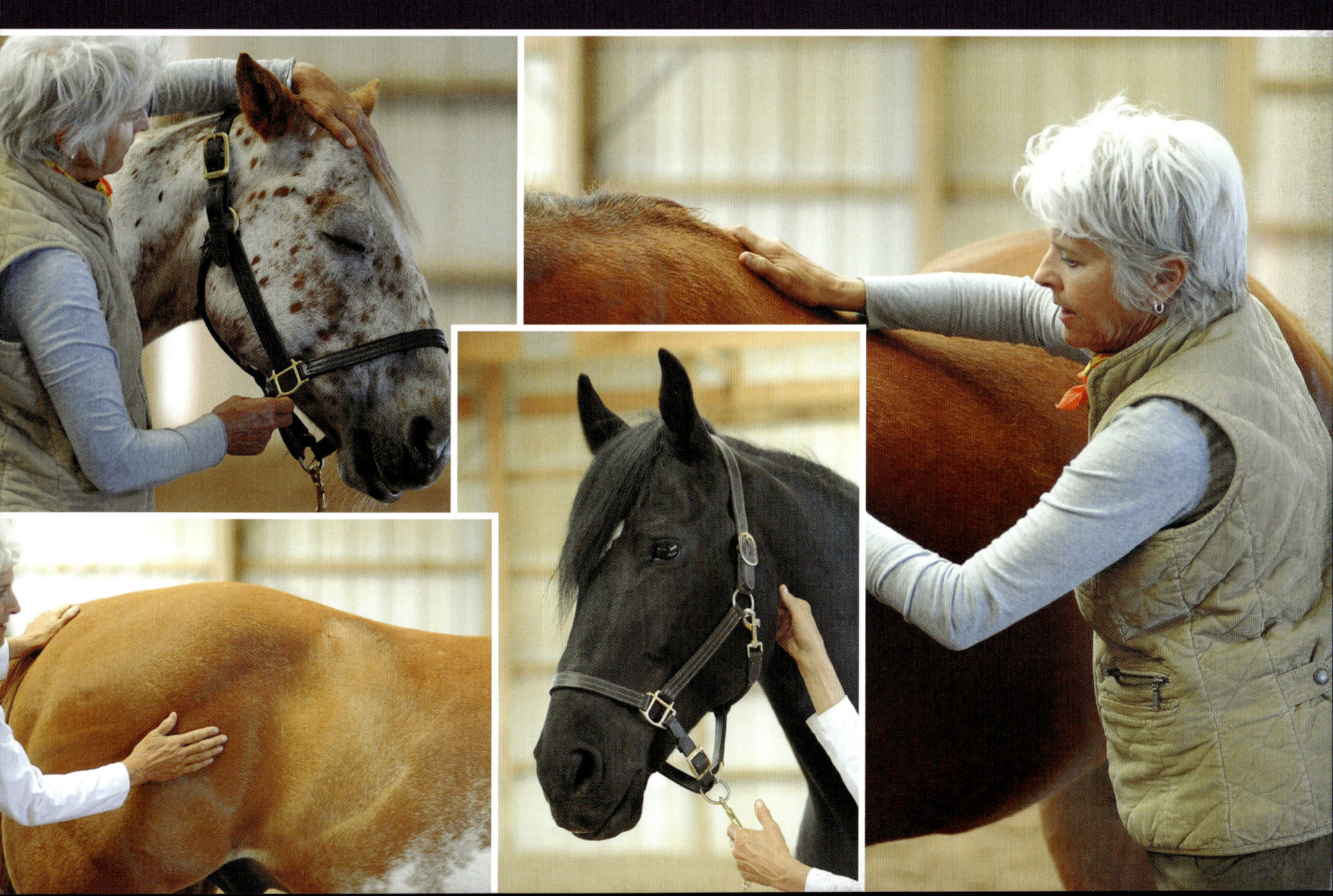

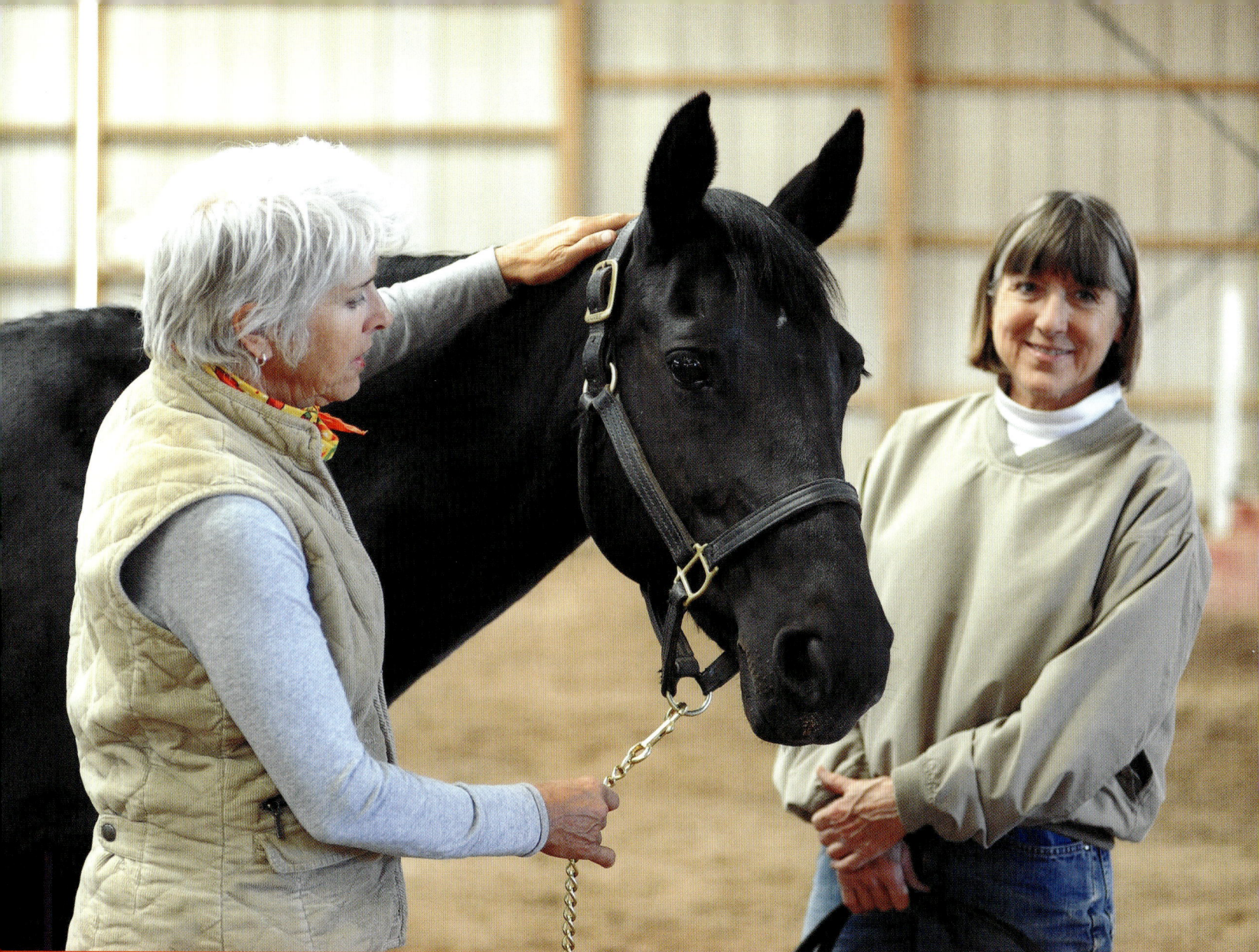

1 | Myofascia
The Body's Internet

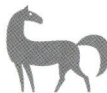

Facts about Myofascia

Myofascia is the gossamer white tissue in the body that connects all the horse's body's parts, including bones, muscles, and all the different body systems. Its unique properties are almost unknown to us, despite its central role in the healthy functioning of all bodies, including humans. As the "internet" of the body, myofascia communicates with all parts instantly, while also giving the horse structure and organization. I use the terms *myofascia*, *fascia*, and *connective tissue* interchangeably throughout this book as I explore this remarkable tissue and how horses transform past limitations from accidents, trauma, and repetitive strain.

Fascia is primarily composed of collagen, elastin, and a polysaccharide gel complex. This combination creates an independent, three-dimensional network of elastic, extremely strong support for the athletic stresses of the horse's body. The collagen has the ability to stiffen and "melt." The elastin allows fascia to both stretch and contract. Fascia is also self-intelligent and self-organizing. Its own fascial layer surrounds every individual organ and muscle inside the horse (figs. 1.1 A & B).

Fascia looks sheer and flimsy, yet it has a very high tensile strength of over 2,000 pounds per inch. When you look at a meat product in its grocery tray, fascia is the filmy, gossamer-white tissue that surrounds

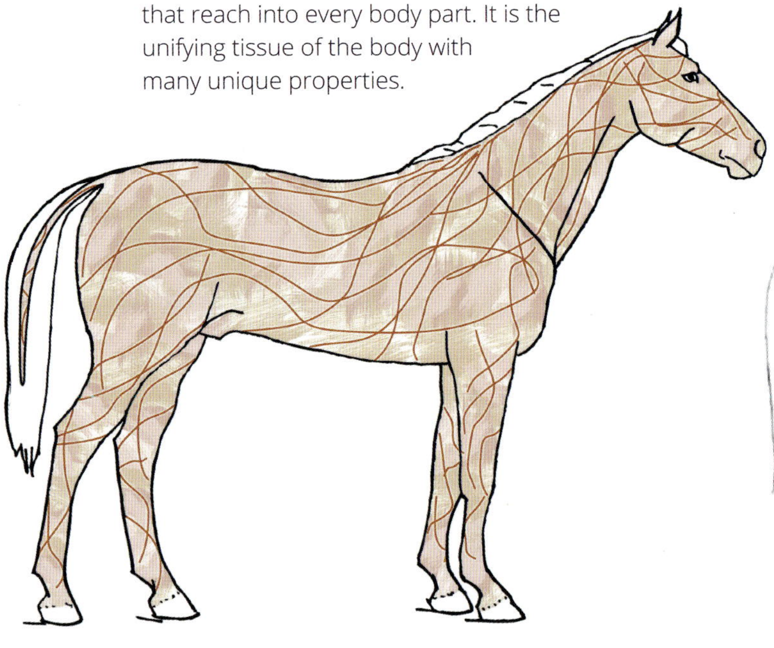

▼ **1.1 A** Horse with art illustrating the flow and gossamer texture of the "internet" of fascia. Fascia is a filmy, flowing tissue with structural items that reach into every body part. It is the unifying tissue of the body with many unique properties.

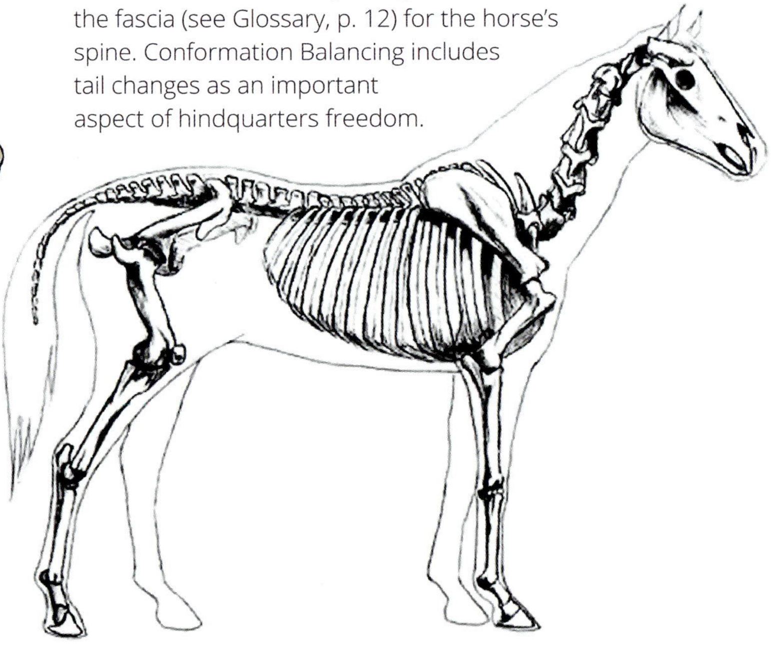

▼ **1.1 B** A drawing of the horse's skeleton, showing the tail. The tail is an important element of the horse's conformation since it often holds many "compensations" related to the fascia (see Glossary, p. 12) for the horse's spine. Conformation Balancing includes tail changes as an important aspect of hindquarters freedom.

muscle and holds it to the bone. It doesn't seem strong, until you try to pull one part from another. This flimsy tissue is usually cut with a sharp knife because it can't be pulled apart. This paradox of fragility yet extreme strength is part of the fascia miracle. Even bones are mineralized fascia.

The internet-like aspects of fascia conduct bioelectric signals to every part of the body in the web. Fascia is a shock absorber due to its collagen, elastic, and gel composition. It is a tension sensor as it conducts micro-currents throughout the body. It also stores water and functions in hydration for the body, which prevents fatigue and toxin buildup. Fascia can organize into scar tissue, knots, or other structural "compensations" for injury. It also participates in the circulatory system's flow of nourishment and fluids. Finally, it is involved with maintaining proper muscle fitness so that all muscles can slide and move freely.

Strain of the fascia also affects all these functions: muscle development; lymphatic function; digestion; meridians; the nervous system; internal organs; and hair quality. Fascial fibers are the anatomical structure that meridians follow, which are the energetic lines developed by the ancient Chinese acupuncture practice.

The self-intelligent fascia organizes itself without intent or conscious direction. A person's warm hand invites the fascia to respond in its own manner. Unlike most approaches to body therapy, fascial change acts independently of patterns. This is an amazingly important detail. Since fascia responds immediately to resolve issues throughout the entire body with self-direction

> "When one tugs at a single thing in nature, he finds it attached to the rest of the world."
> —*John Muir*

and self-intelligence, we don't control its process. In fact, you can be sure that hand contact on fascia will surpass results you planned, as well as accomplishing changes that you don't imagine.

Within an instant of body strain, the entire network of fascia mobilizes to protect the animal. Fascia moves self-intelligently to create solutions helping the horse recover from strain or injury. Fascia's unique properties allow it to hide from the usual diagnostic evaluations, and often show little regarding damage. Pain is seldom associated with tight fascia itself although we know from our human experience that a strain hurts. Medications are temporarily useful in easing or ending pain, but they do not change the fascia or help it organize itself.

The elusive properties of fascia allow it to slip through the cracks of science, but it is now a health and fitness frontier. Myofascial work is one of the myriad holistic ways to progress body health and fitness, along with massage, chiropractic, meridian work, acupuncture, and acupressure. The unique internet-like structure of fascia means that your work with fascia is actually much easier, since you are not searching for tiny points or meridians, or other small areas on the horse. It is an ever-present, organizing tissue that connects all the parts.

The Living Trinity: Body, Emotions, and Spirit

Now that we know some common facts about fascia, let's take a larger view of this amazing body tissue.

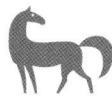

GLOSSARY OF TERMS

Adhesions: The result of long-term or chronic strain, adhesions are fascia that has hardened over time. They can be almost immobile, or wooden in texture. Large areas of adhesions don't move well or cooperate with other body parts.

Compensations: Fascia that thickens to support strain of any sort. Compensations are dispersed throughout the body to retain balance. Because they are thicker, they don't move freely with surrounding tissue. Compensations are found anywhere, and are often not close to where the strain is located. For example, a strain in the right shoulder can have compensating fascia in the left hindquarter.

Conformation Advances: Improvements in the horse's appearance due to freedom of movement.

Dural Tube: The tube of fascia that encases the spine.

Energy Cyst: Tissue that holds memory of trauma. Trauma has stayed in the cells of the fascia and now blocks the energy flow of normal life processes. The term "energy cyst" was developed by Dr. John Upledger, as cited in Soma-Emotional Recall.

Fascia Changes: These can be changes in chemistry when fascia becomes hard and brittle after a strain or injury, or when strain or injury is countered with Conformation Balancing, and the fascia becomes soft, "flowing," and freely moving with the heat of the hand.

Imbalance: A horse cannot show easy movement when he is stiff or has immobile parts of his body. As a result, gaits are awkward and uneven; transitions are difficult; he may stumble often. And he continually injures himself in his environment.

Melt: This describes how stiff and rigid fascia changes under the hand's heat. The tightness of the restricted fascia releases, giving you a "melting" sensation.

Myofascia/Fascia/Connective Tissue: The white, filmy tissue that organizes all body parts. It has high-tensile strength and a random structure. Fascia is composed of elastin, collagen, and a polysaccharide gel complex.

Myofascial Release: Often called MFR, this bodywork method employs handwork to warm and change myofascia (fascia/connective tissue) that has become restricted or tightened from strain or an accident.

Release: An opening, or relaxing, of tight or compressed fascia. This brings pain relief.

Still Point: When the horse's attention focuses inward on fascia changes. The eyes show intense concentration. The Still Point should not be interrupted.

Soma-Emotional Recall: A term developed by Dr. John Upledger and defined in *Craniosacral Therapy* by Upledger and Vredevoogd (Eastland Press, 1983). Tissue, especially connective tissue, is known to have memory. When there is a traumatic event, the energy often enters the body and gets stuck: it walls itself off and blocks the body's natural energy flow. This is also sometimes referred to as an "energy cyst" (see above).

Sacral Juncture: The area where the spine connects to the pelvis. Also referred to as the "sacrum."

Fascia contains a living trinity of body, emotions, and spirit. Fascia's unique role in body structure includes holding emotional memory and consciousness. For the horse, this emotional content is particularly important.

Horses are large animals and our safety depends on their cooperation. When there's an area of emotional trauma trapped in fascia, we'll often find it in a very sensitive area or a place where there is much dense, stuck tissue. As we patiently melt it, the fascia tissue releases with Soma-Emotional Recall, and the horse remembers the accident or problem he experienced. If we stay patiently with his change, he realizes he is safe now and we are helping him recover himself. This improvement in his being impresses the horse and growth comes for him: he now knows that the rider, as a true leader, can help him. We accept the horse's fear as real and help him truly change. This mutual experience brings trust for both horse and rider.

For horses, this new trust is transformative. They lose old anxieties and live, instead, in the present. For riders and people working with horses, this method of progress is incredibly effective and efficient. Imagine, the old anxieties disappear without hundreds of training hours. This Soma-Emotional Recall process is also available for people, usually with a MFR (myofascial release) therapist. However, this book focuses on our important friend, the horse. The horse's progressive changes are the stories here.

If this body/emotional/spiritual process of fascia is mysterious, we are even more astounded when we realize how little we usually know about fascia. Yet the paradox is that, like the internet or electricity, though we know little about fascia, we completely rely on it. An irritation or injury entering the network of fascia affects our and the horse's whole body with referred pain or restricted movement called "compensations." These compensations spread everywhere in the horse. A fingertip touch not only accesses the body part touched, but also reaches the fascia in all parts. A "jaw touch" brings fascia changes to the horse's hindquarters, as well as to a million—or billion—other locations.

> The self-intelligent fascia presents an internet for us to explore; one touch spreads changes throughout the horse, as needed.

This instant change is why fascia is not only highly efficient and comprehensive, it is also extremely progressive. This is why an injury or strain might seem unimportant, but it causes major loss of competence later. The buildup of repeated strain from any riding discipline, injury, or life condition for the horse eventually limits the horse's performance ability, or even makes it impossible for the horse to continue. When all the parts are connecting with balance, all goes well. But when fascia has become stuck, whole areas of the horse are only partially accessible. This loss may not show immediately following an injury, but the body's response becomes slower and less competent. In this book, you learn how Conformation Balancing facilitates change that releases stuck areas, and allows the entire being to restructure itself.

Like the internet web, each body site brings a universe of connectivity. As we touch the horse, fascia changes itself, and remarkably, it is not even necessary for us to focus intent for the change. An example of this pervasive importance of fascia is the gurgling and

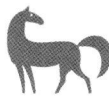

rumblings of the horse's organs when we are working on his skin. If these amazing properties of fascia seem impossible, consider how animals and humans healed themselves for millions of years. They lay down and rested with others for company, and moved occasionally while their body's tissue performed the recovery. Today, we are rediscovering fascia because of the high demands of the horse-sport world and the long-term training investments made in our horses.

Conformation Balancing is not achieved through medication, diet, exercise, or even massage. Instead, fascia responds to temperature for its change. While it may not seem scientific, hand heat brings precisely the correct heat for fascia changes. This emphasis on hand-temperature change brings up another common misunderstanding about injured and strained body tissue. The body's reaction to strain with heat ensures that the fascia stays elastic and supportive to the strain, helping keep the body balanced, instead of the strained area hardening and becoming numb.

Although the common practice is to treat strain and inflammation with ice or cold, fascia does not respond progressively to cold. Cold makes fascia lose elasticity, and the horse's collagen hardens more quickly into adhesions. Cold temperatures actually hasten the hardening and numbing of fascial tissue. The swelling goes down and the heat dissipates, but fascia's self-healing action is stopped and frozen. The injured area may move more quickly again because the horse is numbed to the strain, but this numbness actually deceives the horse and rider into further injury, as well as many more compensations later.

So, how does this remarkable tissue change under strain and accidental injury? Due to its remarkable properties, it doesn't snap or break like a bone. It immediately builds many cross-hatching fibers in all directions around the area of strain, as well as faraway areas that help hide the strain for the horse (figs. 1.2 A & B).

At first, these areas are warmer and larger as the fascia adds support. Eventually, they return to a more normal size and temperature, but the composition of the fascia changes. Over time, instead of flowing easily, it hardens into stiff fibers and lumps called "adhesions." Adhesions are hard, tight, and, sometimes, crunchy. These adhesions grow stiffer with time and eventually feel wooden. Many of us know about frozen-shoulder

Normal Fascia

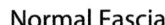

A

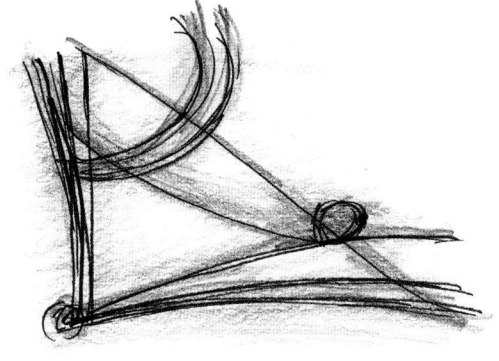

▶ **1.2 A & B** Normal fascia compared with "compensated" fascia (with adhesions). Notice the rigidity in the adhesion art in B. This stiffness is why fluid movement is lost for the horse with "compensations," and also why compensations hurt.

Fascia with Adhesions

B

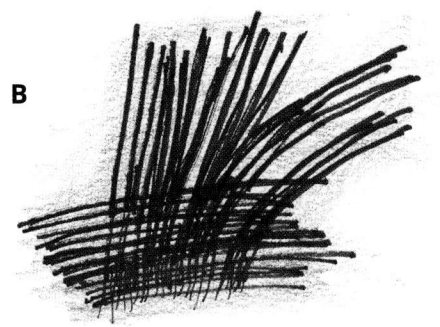

syndrome where our entire shoulder is completely stuck, unable to move.

Intense injury brings more adhesions than simple strains, and they block movement in muscle groups as well as circulation of blood and fluids. Soreness, pain, and restricted range of motion all result from adhesions. As the number of adhesions grows, whole areas of the horse's body are affected and limited by them. We call these physical limitations "compensations." Compensations are how the horse's body hides the injury by using other areas to support the weak, strained area. This compensation behavior assures the horse that he looks fit to any nearby predator.

Eventually, the adhesions also tighten whole groups of joints and muscles, then the horse is restricted and loses various abilities: the fascia that surrounds each muscle controls and contains it. When the fascia around a muscle is pulled tight, the muscle cannot grow or expand with work. Compensations travel to the deeper layers of fascia around the internal organs, causing poor digestion or disruption in heart or lung capacity. An injury that seems to have healed has actually brought intense difficulties for the horse, and he can't tell us about them.

These stiff adhesions seem impossible to change at first. Yet, as we use warm hands to melt the hard tissue, the stiff tissue softens and melts just when it seems that nothing will change. The fascia responds by releasing heat, which was stored energy, from the dense tight fascia. This heat release can almost burn your hands.

Many horses allow very deep, old adhesions to change in the very first session. The ear, poll, jaw, and dock of the tail are often the site of very old stuck connective tissue. The shoulders also invite our continual

fascial changes. Proceed at the horse's pace—there is always far more progress than you can imagine in the billions of "body net sites" with one touch. Often, you must work with the less sensitive areas on the horse first, until trust in the change is established.

There's a simple experiment to test how fascia changes on yourself. Find a spot where you have lost range of motion, stiffness or an old injury; perhaps, you have a sore spot on the side of a knee, elbow, or hip, or where it hurts. Then, place your hand on the area, allowing hand heat to soften it. This may take a few minutes or longer depending how cold your hands are or how stuck the tissue is. The hand must be warm enough to melt the stuck area.

With patience, you'll feel the change, even if slight at first. As you keep your warm hand on the area, you'll begin to feel more change in the spot and maybe in another area of your body. If you do this for at least 15 minutes or longer, changes happen. This is an easy way to discover how amazingly effective fascial change is for the body. As you practice, discover how the fascia changes spread through your entire body self-intelligently. Notice sensations in your ankle from arm contact. Each body has its own way of compensating, but the patterns surface quickly with continued practice.

Conformation Is Organized by Fascia

Conformation is not only the horse's inborn natural ability and structural appearance, it is also his ability and structure in real time. Conformation structure includes how the horse stands, how efficiently he uses his body, and whether all the parts are functioning completely. The horse's entire being is included in conformation. When

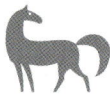

a horse is born genetically well balanced and capable, yet loses his ability by three years of age, he is no longer perceived by us, or himself, as a fit and capable horse. The athletic gifts of good conformation become lost to him and us. He knows he should be able to do his work, but he can't. He's confused by this loss of ability. There may be little or no active pain, yet he can't move well. This lack of fitness then brings him anxiety and defensiveness: insecurity is extremely dangerous for a prey animal, which is why imbalance and cellular memory of injury causes so much difficulty for him (fig. 1.3).

We humans are the same (although we're at the top of the food chain these days). We all know of a rider who has "lost her nerve" after an accident, or perhaps it's an athlete who has the ability yet cannot access her gifts fully. This is the result of the body's cellular memory, or Soma-Emotional Recall, which we have defined as trauma held in the fascial tissue itself. While science often ignores emotional energy as unimportant, it is indeed a factor in fascial health.

Now you see how a horse's conformation is affected by the state of his fascia. As areas of strain or injury progress, whole sections of his body lose their shape and function. Shoulders have a "hollow" look. Hips lose their muscle. The neck almost wastes away due to the compression of tight fascia. This overall slow compression due to a single-strain event progresses eventually to a place where the horse "just can't do that anymore." A left lead at the canter can't happen. Or, collection goes from being "difficult" to do, to work we don't attempt. A once-fit horse becomes consistently lame.

A balanced, fit horse can competently move through extreme stresses such as jumping or racing, but a horse with compensations cannot even stand square. Worst of all, the adhesions continue to tighten, creating even more compensation patterns. He has no way to be comfortable again. Drugs may dull the pain, but they won't restore movement.

This slow but progressive loss of fascial balance throughout the horse's body seems to appear suddenly. One day, we realize our horse doesn't look good. He's unable to easily stand square, his shoulders and hind end aren't muscled well, and his back dips. He's hard to tack up because he hurts. Correct lead changes are impossible. We don't canter anymore. He is inconsistent in his performance. Finally, the horse is cranky and

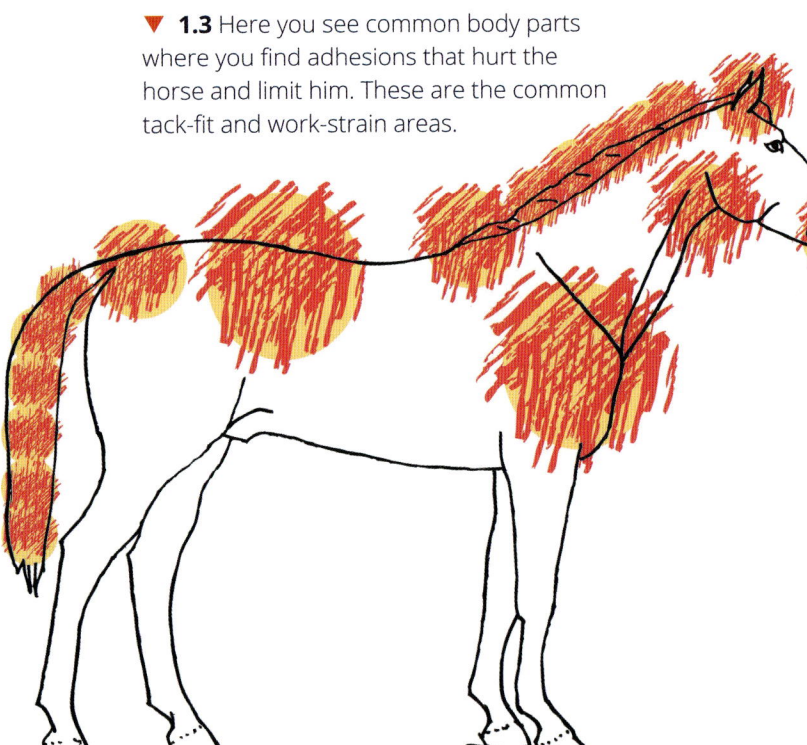

▼ **1.3** Here you see common body parts where you find adhesions that hurt the horse and limit him. These are the common tack-fit and work-strain areas.

irritable. We are not having much fun together. Is a new horse the answer, we ask ourselves? If we love or even like our horse, we tend to accept the limits and learn to do less with him. The cycle of looking for "fixes" begins.

There's a solution to this loss of fitness. Just as we know people who have recovered full fitness from all kinds of accidents, the horse can recover, too. The Conformation Balancing process leads to dramatic improvements when we follow the visual clues and learn to look carefully at our horse's shape and stance. We look past good breeding and pleasant features as our eyes learn to see, and as our hands feel his body, we find areas of hardness, stiffness, and pain. These are the blockages to easy movement and full muscle development. For example, hidden pockets of tightness prevent a shoulder from building sufficient muscle to fill out high, hollow withers. The visual signs of a "used-up horse" are nearly always temporary problems.

A Vital Aspect: Soma-Emotional Recall

As we now know, nearly every horse experiences strain and injury. Young horses, in particular, have injuries that lodge in their fascia, carrying the trauma of an event. Perhaps they had a bad loading situation, or an accident involving a fence in the pasture. A foal may have landed on his head at birth or rough social play caused a head injury. These kinds of events bring fear that lodges in the fascia and become an anxiety factor for the horse when similar situations or pressures arrive. We call these "energy cysts" since they hold old traumatic energy and emotions, much like Post-Traumatic Stress Disorder (PTSD) in soldiers or other people doing dangerous work.

THE KEY TO AWARENESS AND HEALTH

Consciousness, which often seems a mental property, is actually awareness. Expanded awareness also results from opening fascial space in the body. The point, in a nutshell, is when compression in fascia releases, the movement of the spreading and expanding fascia brings awareness and health. Movement is health for the body. Balance is health for the body. This is true for all beings.

These energy cysts eventually debilitate the horse's conformation—and personality. When the accident happens early in his life, the horse never achieves mental balance and lasting success in his work. This is the mysterious cause of the many well-bred horses who lapse into non-productive lives. Handsome horses with head bangs and hind-end dents from kicks are often in this non-productive category.

Conformation Balancing is a simple solution for many of these traumas. When you put your hand on an affected area where the horse has an energy cyst and stay on it, letting the fascia fully "melt," a Still Point occurs for the horse as he feels the cellular memory for the old unpleasant event surface. The horse gets an inward look with a soft, unfocused expression. He chews slowly and blinks. His muzzle trembles. This is a major change for him. He revisits the entire event, the

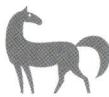

"held" emotional energy cyst opens, and the old "stuck" energy moves out of the fascial cells.

This is an energetic change, but it is not "energy work." The change results from fascial cell release. We do indeed use our hand heat to initiate the change, but it is the heat temperature that does the work, not our intention or personal energy focusing on the horse.

These amazing fascia changes are part physical chemistry, part emotional therapy, and part spiritual transformation. The horse truly changes. The old fear dissolves when there are enough fascia changes. Sometimes, more than one releasing change is needed. It takes what it takes. At times, there is so much stored in the fascia that many hand contacts are required to completely transform that old panic experience. This process is a miracle for the horse.

> The horse's comfort and agreement is vital.

We watch carefully for that inward look in the horse's eye, and stay with the horse without disturbing his experience of this inside change. The Still Point is where conscious acceptance for his own experience brings him freedom from the trauma. His entire fascial network receives the message that this terrible event has been processed. No fear is needed now to warn the horse of more danger.

A horse trapped in anxiety from old trauma, damaging training procedures, or an accident can't respond fully to the present when this cellular memory is active. Not every behavior problem with a horse is the result of fascial strain, but a high percentage of difficult behaviors and fearful responses show these cellular sources. After an injury, the horse's inborn conformation often changes within a few years or less.

Looking around, you can see examples of well-bred horses that don't look "well built," so something has gone wrong in the "internet" of fascia. Like a website that doesn't load properly, or has missing pieces, the horse's body isn't functioning well. For example, in addition to the obvious strained shoulder, his entire fascial "network" is tightened from the injury. So, while you might see a single injury, if indeed you even know about it, the horse's physical and emotional experience of the injury is very complex and much deeper in impact.

The horses in the photos that follow show how horses feel a Still Point or conscious change of the fascia (figs. 1.4–1.9). These inner-focus moments must not be interrupted in order to bring successful change.

As I noted early on, the horse's head is a high priority. Headstalls, longeing, and tying can bring accidents and strain for the horse's head balance. When head-balancing, we repeat our hand contact as often as he'll accept it. Often, poll contact or in-mouth contact lasts many minutes before it brings the horse to a lick-and-chew signal. It may take 15 minutes or more for Still Points to release completely. Patience is rewarded. These head-injury problems are a dark secret of the horse world.

The truth is that a horse with compensations is often numb in many places and can't respond to the rider. He can't feel his hind end enough to round it. Or, he can't feel his ribs enough on one side to yield to an aid. He really wants to respond correctly because his entire genetic blueprint is for a specific skill, whether dressage, cutting, jumping, or other discipline. So, the talented, elite horse that loves excellence and craves our approval spends days without free expression of his abilities. His frustration becomes immense. His body hurts, thus his defense is to simply reject the rider and the work to save his own life.

Many horses have over 500 years of highly intentional breeding. Horses are bred for performance, temperament, intelligence, character, and color, to name a few genetic goals. When the horse's entire genetic makeup is frustrated by the progression of small and hidden compensations, the horse is depressed and, sometimes, angry with his rider for requesting what he can't do. However well-intentioned, when the rider continually asks for what the horse can't access, the horse mentally hits a wall, perhaps putting the rider into a wall!

Often, in this work, the horse will direct us through his willingness to experience specific changes. He directs us to areas he wants to change first, and shows us how deep we can go. When the horse moves us on from a critical area, we discover later that other changes were necessary for the larger ones to succeed.

As this work with the fascia progresses and integrates, we see conformation improve: Toplines balance. Necks lengthen, withers rise, muzzles realign, tails lift and plume. We see "nicks" in withers disappear. We see dips in the sacral area vanish as the hindquarters become balanced again. The results may come quickly in one session, though sometimes they take four sessions—or even a year—in cases of multi-compensations for a serious injury.

Conformation Balancing brings a new appearance for the horse and a return of the horse's fitness. Often, the horse advances far past his original ability. Many accidents limiting horses occur when they are young and, as mentioned, we don't know the injury occurred.

So the horse's limits often begin at a young age. As we find the limits and clear them, the horse's athletic abilities bloom.

These profound advances excite the rider. The horse feels this delight and a new kind of relationship begins. As our journey with fascia unfolds, we see the consciousness of the horse change with many Still Points. This becomes a revelation, which you'll see many times throughout this book.

Bella: Beginning with the Ears

An example of a horse promptly accepting fascial balancing was a black Welsh Arabian mare that had been ear-twitched as a foal. Bella could barely tolerate her ears being touched, and her owner had great difficulty putting on a headstall or halter. In the mare's first session, we focused on her right ear, sliding the hand up very softly and holding the ear as if it were a baby bird—clear up to the tip. The owner watched in astonishment as the mare's eyes showed complete acceptance and recognition of the fascia changes she was experiencing. She stood completely still and received connective-tissue change in her ear for over 40 minutes. Following the head and poll changes in this session, Bella accepted the halter easily. This was an immediate, one-session change.

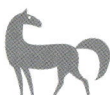

STILL POINT EXAMPLES

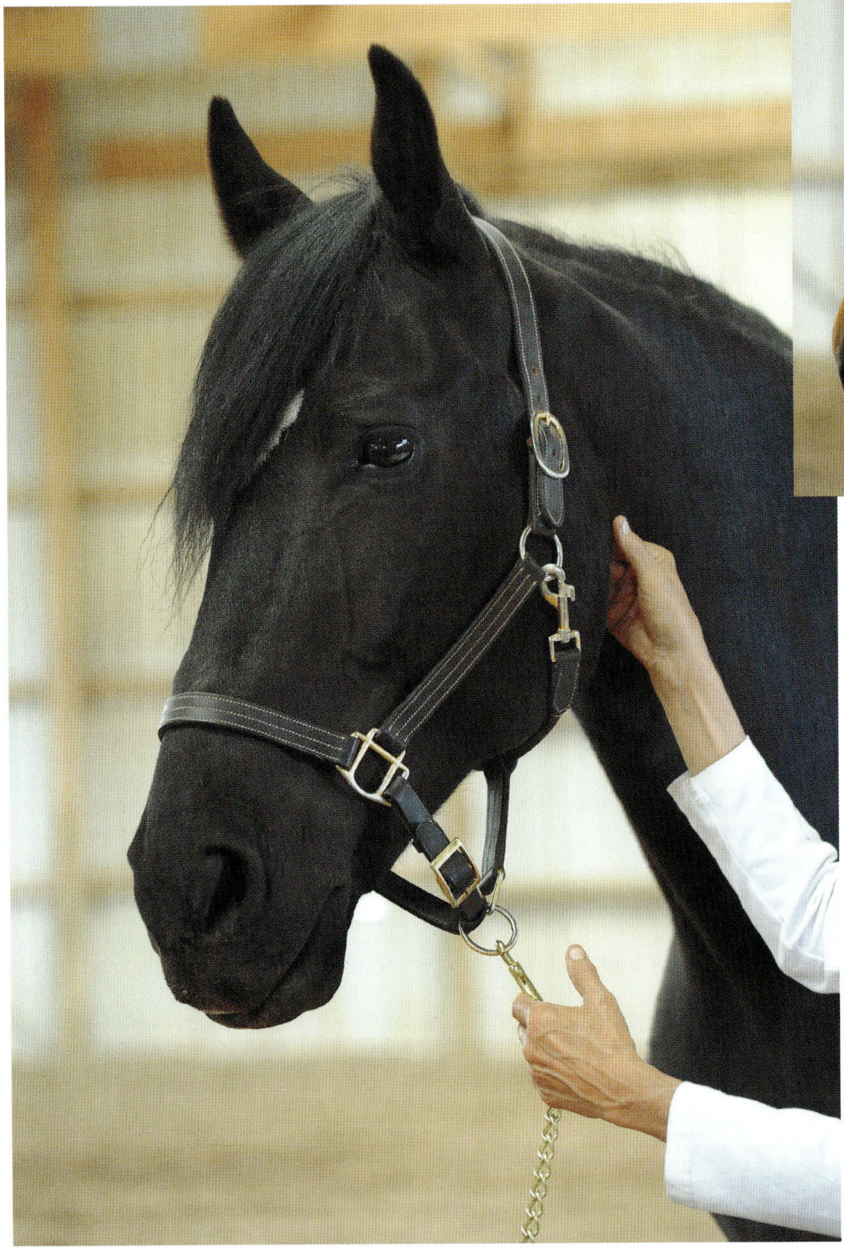

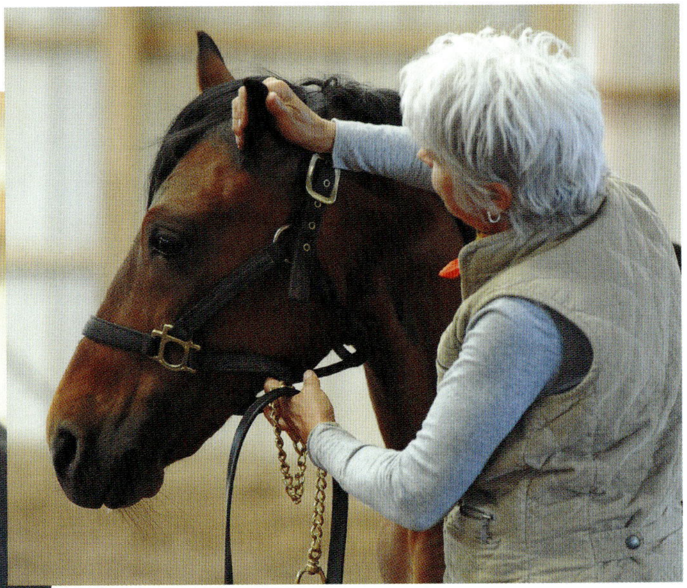

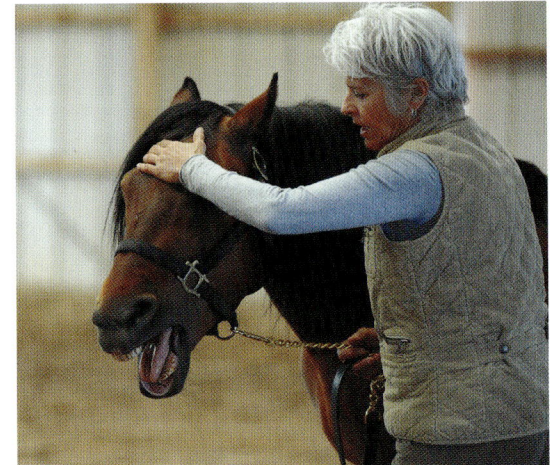

▲ **1.5** Samson, a Paso Fino, intently focuses on his ear changes (see p. 63). The ear is a crucial area for Conformation Balancing, especially since tack fits against the fascia around the ears.

▲ **1.6** Samson expresses change release by yawning while he enjoys his head balancing (see p. 80). Other balancing change cues include blinking, sighing, twitching, trembling, breath exhaling, and other reactions of relief.

▲ **1.4** Beau is in a deep Still Point as he receives a jaw-release change (see p. 64). There is no restraint and my hand contact is soft. My hand is not pushing.

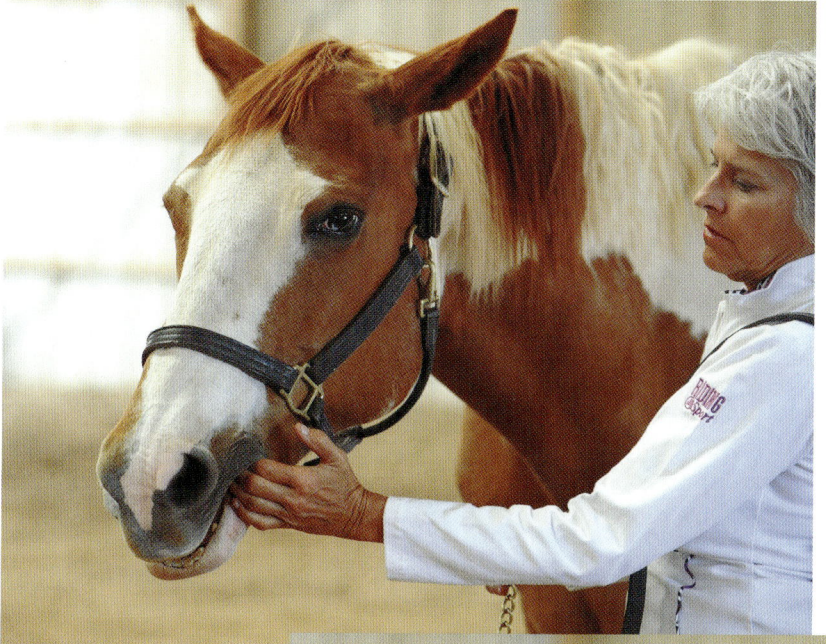

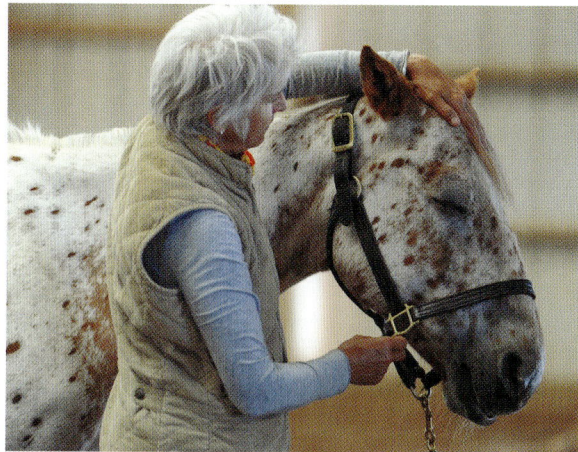

▲ **1.8** Remy is deep in a Still Point as his poll changes with balancing (see p. 80). This simple change often resolves a lot of anxiety for the horse, allowing him to be receptive without old fears controlling his behavior.

▲ **1.7** Scout enjoys a Still Point in this in-mouth release. Here, I'm resting my fingers on the jaw, in the space where the bit sits, gently. My position here allows Scout to create the balance he needs.

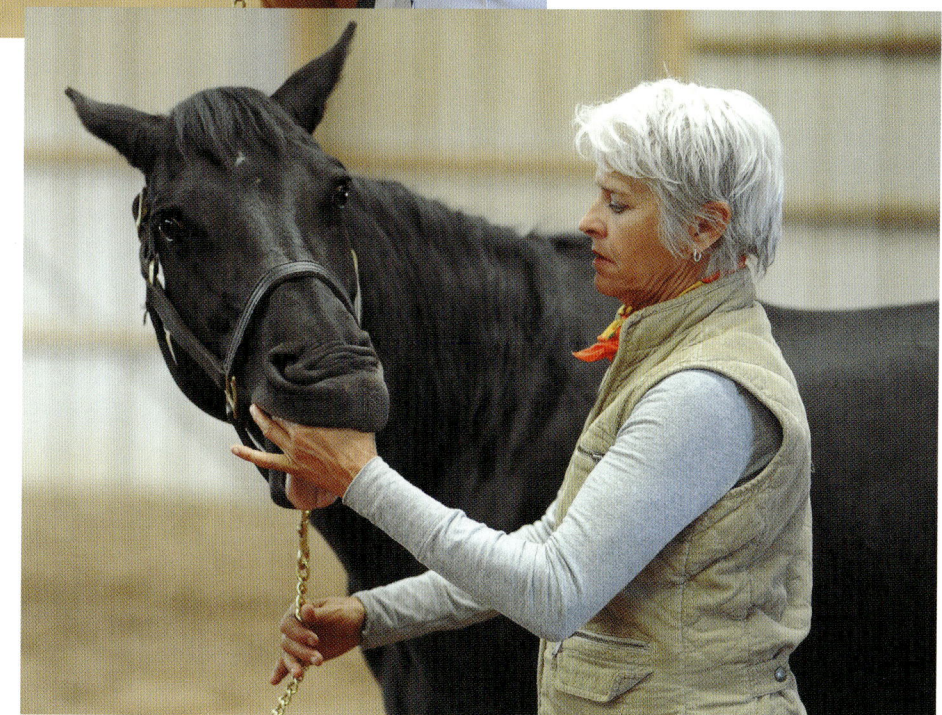

◄ **1.9** Here, Jet enjoys a front lip change (see p. 86). The web of the index finger and thumb are up against the horse's gums. This balances the entire spine as well as his head.

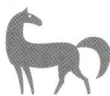

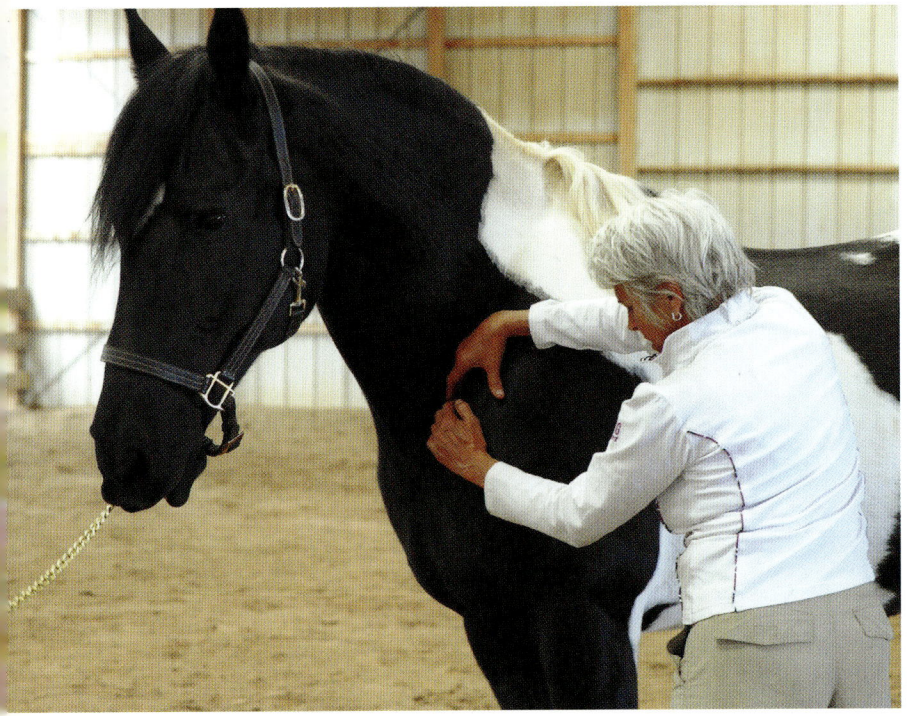

▲ **1.10** The horse's eyes show his approval when I'm working intimately with his body.

To make progress with your horse's fitness, you practice and follow the horse's cues. Use the conformation inventory outlined in Part I to assess your horse and then work with the methods in Part II to solve your horse's particular issues.

The techniques presented grow more effective with sensitive hands able to read the tissue to find compensations and strain. Big changes are effected in small amounts of time. When years of stuck tissue, imbalance, and pain exist, the horse needs your patience as he opens to the change and unwinds his anxiety regarding large stiff areas such as shoulders and hips. Repetition brings reward. So, when there are large stiff areas on your horse, don't despair. A "breakthrough" melt in the hard, stiff fascia will come and lead the way to faster progress.

Conformation Balancing Is Not About You

Working with horses' fascia is very intimate. You stand very close and handle them in sensitive places on a routine basis (fig. 1.10). For the professional, the circumstances are always changing, and the horses are often new. With consistent good judgment, the horse will approve your work. Attention to your body position and environment is vital in safe work. Most importantly, you do not insist on meeting your own goals; you always agree to end the hand contact when the horse is "full."

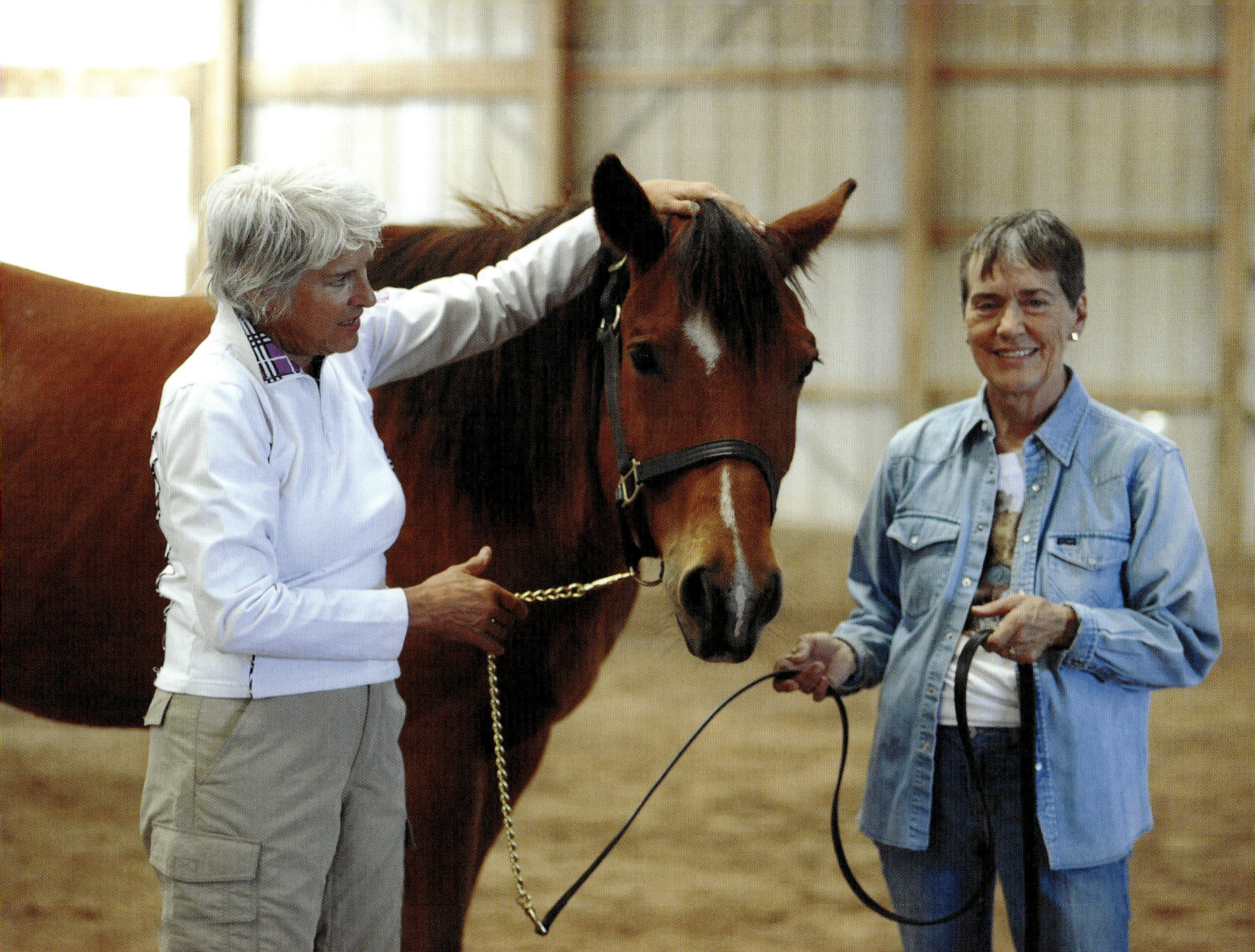

2 | How the Horse Looks and Moves

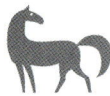

Conformation

Let's investigate conformation. It is defined in the dictionary as the structure or outline of a being determined by the arrangement of its parts. Horse people know that a horse's conformation is far more than structure or outline. It also includes how a horse moves, plus that almost indefinable quality of how the horse organizes himself, and his "talent" at being a horse. It's the "I know it when I see it" recognition. You can usually recognize a well-built horse—even with variations such as age, breed difference, and athletic development. (Breed registries define conformation for registered horses according to their own standards.)

Conformation is also a tool for everyone involved with horses to recognize athletic and physical assets. However, I will leave the halter-class criteria and horse-show definitions to those industry experts because the focus of the work here is to address the authenticity and comfort of the horse's present structure for him.

So, in the work here, "conformation" identifies areas for balancing fascia and indicates the horse's talents. The overall look of the horse shows you where you can begin to help him. Imbalances show up in how the horse fits together. Here, you will be learning how to use conformation as a healing tool, not a halter-class evaluation.

How to See Conformation

A general rule is first to look at the overall shape of the horse then observe larger and smaller areas to see how these fit together. For example, a sturdy horse with small hindquarters shows you an imbalance. When sections of the horse's body are smaller or lighter looking, the lighter section is usually considered an imbalance; it makes the neighboring section look larger. The smaller area is an imbalance resulting from an injury.

Strained or injured areas have compressed fascia, which prevents muscles from building properly. This imbalance affects the entire authentic structure of the horse and changes his movement. The larger area nearby, or even on the other end of the horse, supports the injured area. For example, when the shoulders are strained, they unbalance the horse—they will not look sufficient for his size or build, or his head might look very large since his neck is undeveloped.

The best way to practice these conformation observations is to look at many horses and begin noticing this "fitting together" of the parts, and their proportion under the topline. When practicing, be sure you immediately discount the idea that the horse isn't well built due to his genetics. Genetics are often blamed for how horses look. You want to learn to see the horse as he is without getting stuck on "he has these conformation defects because of the type of horse he is."

Let's practice. You see a horse with a large barrel, a thin undeveloped neck, and high bony withers. The horse does not look appealing. Your observation tells you the horse is not well built, yet perhaps the horse is very well bred. So, how does this happen?

The horse's body reveals all the strains and stresses in his life. He starts out fit, perhaps, but then spends years in side-reins or doing quick full stops that tighten his back and sacrum. Then his shoulders tighten so

> Always look at how the horse fits together.

much that his neck muscle deteriorates. His back loses tone and his barrel becomes a potbelly. He looked "good" until his youthful vigor was gone. Now, at 16 years, he looks like an old horse.

This story is common in the horse world. This loss of conformational balance seems to come exactly when the training has progressed and the horse is an asset to us. We've both finally learned enough, but now the horse can't do things. We lament this, if we can see it clearly. These kinds of common imbalances in horses that last for years lead to unbalanced conformation, soundness problems, lack of ability, and anxiety. We lose our best friend too soon!

Let's return to looking at a horse with one part smaller than the other parts. The horse looks out of balance—the smaller, weaker-looking section doesn't look strong enough to keep up. You start in your search for the injury in the smaller areas, the dips and hard areas on the horse's body. With practice, you can repeatedly see the truth of a horse's history in his conformation. When your eyes see even more details, the movement and structure possibilities of the horse become facts, not projections. Smooth, flowing gaits come from a flowing body structure (fig. 2.1).

Classical conformation shows the three parts of the horse as:

1. Nose to withers

2. Barrel

3. Hindquarters

Each of the three parts is equal in "balanced" conformation. The three parts of the horse are a beginning in-

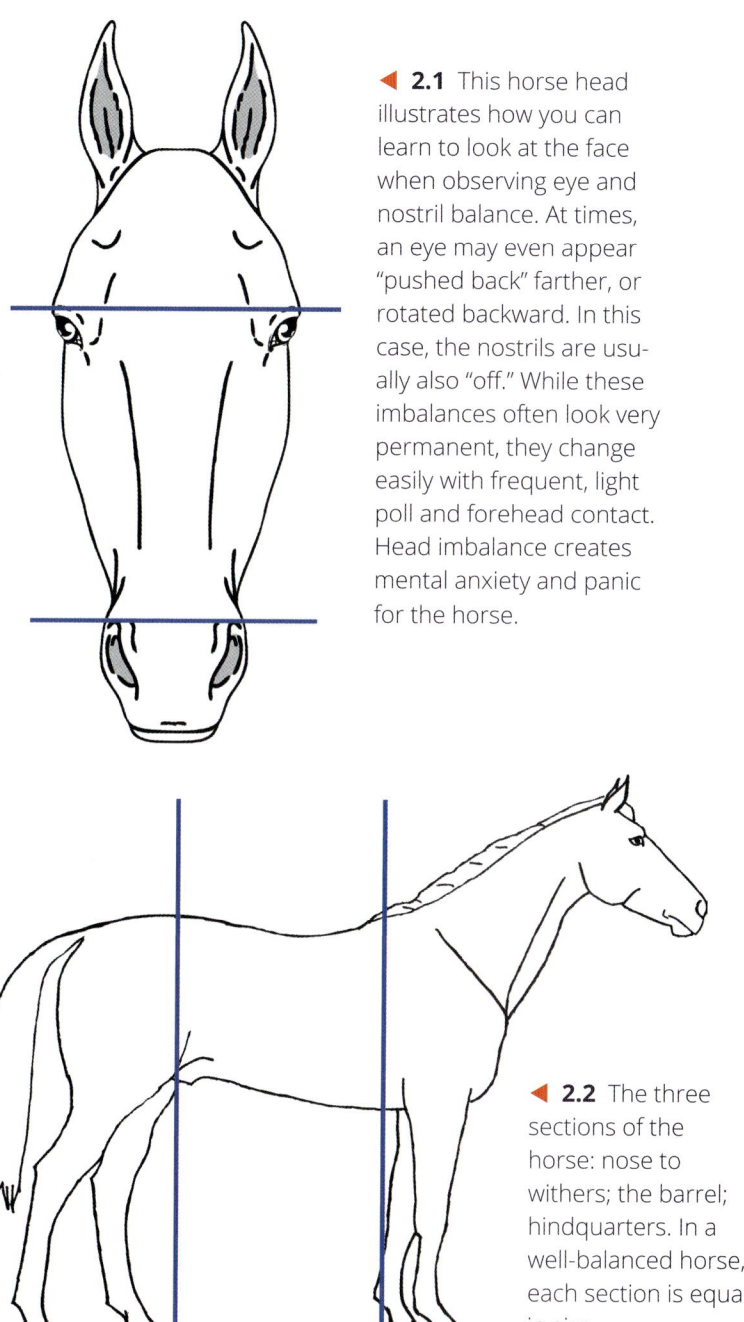

◄ **2.1** This horse head illustrates how you can learn to look at the face when observing eye and nostril balance. At times, an eye may even appear "pushed back" farther, or rotated backward. In this case, the nostrils are usually also "off." While these imbalances often look very permanent, they change easily with frequent, light poll and forehead contact. Head imbalance creates mental anxiety and panic for the horse.

◄ **2.2** The three sections of the horse: nose to withers; the barrel; hindquarters. In a well-balanced horse, each section is equal in size.

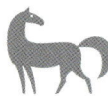

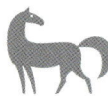

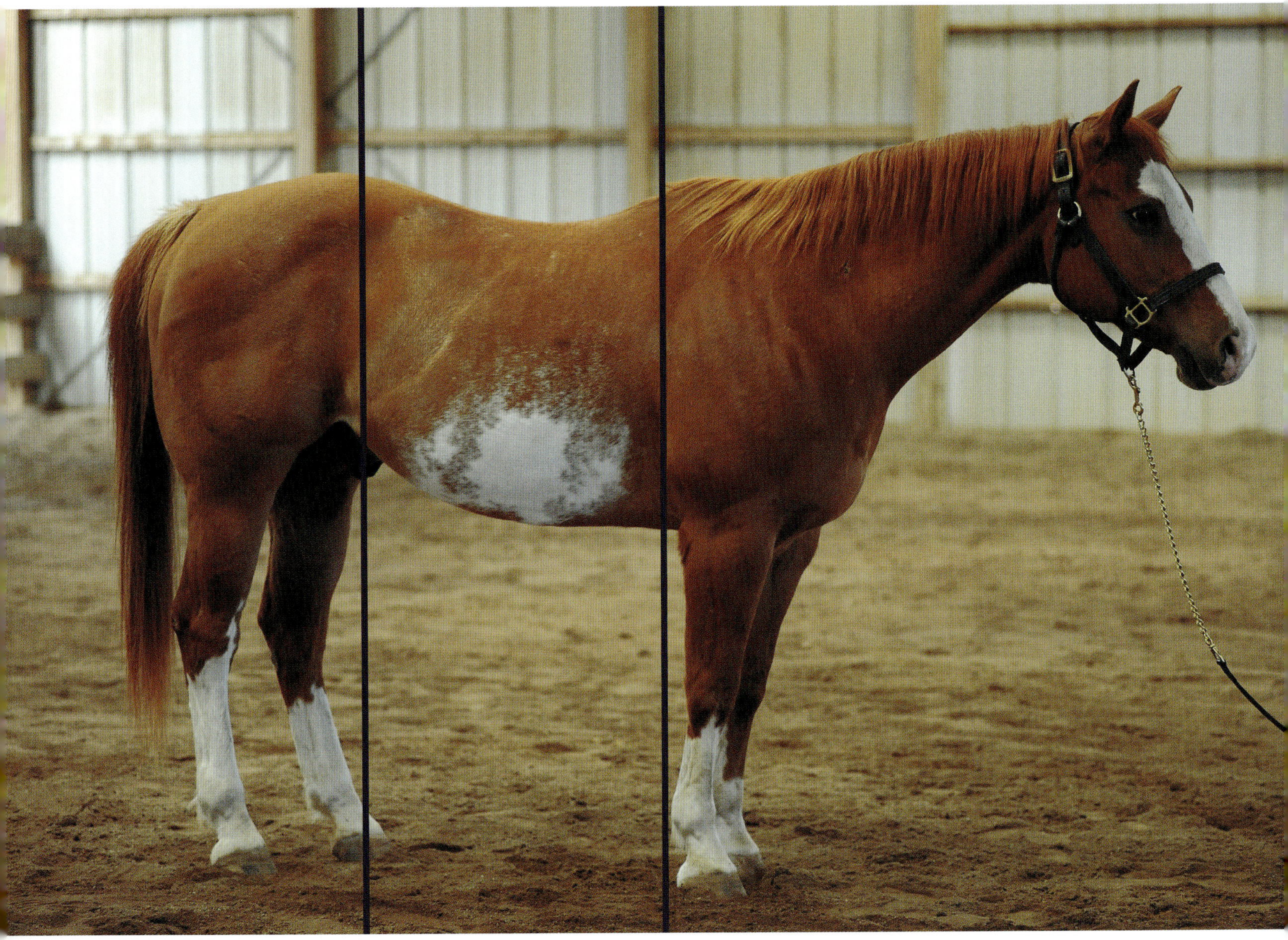

▲ **2.3** Every horse is different; this horse is a good example of a balanced conformation. Notice that each section is nearly equal in size. Differences in age, breed, and work create variations in the sections. "Balanced" conformation does not mean "best" conformation. Each horse is unique and has his own gifts.

ventory for athletic assets. Many talented horses do not show three balanced parts in their conformation. Some horses turn an imbalance into a useful gift. However, a variation in the size of these three sections often indicates that the horse's body has been strained.

This overall view of the horse's three parts is a practical guide, not a rigid format to dismiss horses with unique structures.

How to Assess Conformation

From a distance of about 8 yards, look at the horse. Notice three sections: nose to withers; the barrel; hindquarters. Use your hand or a card to block parts while evaluating the sections. These three sections show a balanced horse when they are nearly equal in size (figs. 2.2 & 2.3).

Balanced Conformation

- A balanced stance is even and "in the box."

- Topline flows without bumps, low areas, or notches.

- Tail carriage is "plumed" or free-flowing.

- Parts of the horse fit together smoothly.

- The horse stands at ease with a peaceful expression.

Imbalanced Conformation

- A "nick" or divot in the neck near the withers.

- Thin neck with no crest.

- Very high withers coupled with undeveloped shoulders.

- A dip in the sacral/loin area.

- A "pot belly" showing on an actively ridden horse.

- A raised backbone without muscle protection.

- An "off" stance where the horse seldom stands square.

- Undeveloped hindquarters.

The Topline

The topline guides your view of conformation (fig. 2.4). As its name suggests, the topline is the visual line that you see tracing along the top of the horse's body. If you look at the horse against a blue sky or other solid visual background, it's easier to see this topline. The topline reveals obvious dips and lumps, as well as showing healthy tissue contrasted with tight, drawn tissue. We usually know if we like the horse's topline and find it attractive or not.

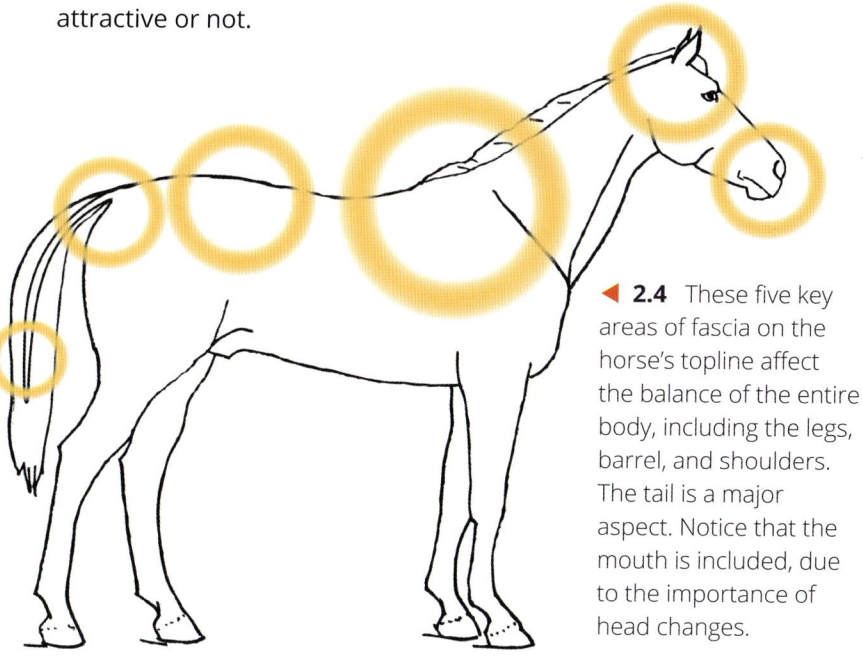

◀ **2.4** These five key areas of fascia on the horse's topline affect the balance of the entire body, including the legs, barrel, and shoulders. The tail is a major aspect. Notice that the mouth is included, due to the importance of head changes.

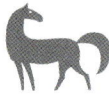

The topline includes the muzzle and follows up his nose, over the poll, along the neck and withers, the back, loins, over his rump and down the tail. A well-balanced topline includes a crested neck, muscled withers, and a sacral/loin/croup area free of lumps or dips. A freely flowing tail is also part of a well-balanced topline. The topline flows on a balanced, fit horse ending in a plumed tail, which shows freedom of hindquarters movement.

When you look at the topline on horses and you

Remember: The horse's body is like the weather. It can change. Notice what "jumps out" visually, today.

see all sorts of dips, lumps and hollows, it's confusing. You don't want to harshly judge the horse, but the visuals don't add up correctly to the horse's history. As mentioned in the last chapter, what happened to the horse often drastically changes how he looks and moves. Often, talented, conscientiously bred horses look quite average in appearance—the process of deterioration in quality horses happens in as little as a year's time. This kind of strain or accident history always shows in every horse.

But, what if you look at your horse and he seems just fine? You see no fear, no bony withers, or hollows. Nothing obvious appears to tell you he's unbalanced. You may be the fortunate rider of a balanced horse with good conformation. Congratulations!

However, many of us look at our horses and see room for improvement. Or maybe your horse looks good, but he doesn't work consistently well. There are also many subtle clues to "stuck" fascia, and as you look at your horse carefully, you'll begin to identify what you're actually seeing. I'm listing here clues to imbalance, both behavioral and visual:

FASCIA LAYERS

Let's review the fascia layers that structure conformation's visual form, even more than genetics or training:

• **Fascia Layer 1:** Directly under the skin. It fits like pantyhose, or long underwear. This layer is the most accessible.

• **Fascia Layer 2:** Organizes the organs, blood vessels, bones, and muscles. Strains in this layer compromise the muscles; this middle fascial internet layer also tightens around the internal organs causing difficult digestive processes or colic. This layer connects all the parts together.

• **Fascia Layer 3:** This deepest layer of fascia surrounds the spinal cord and brain. This layer is the purpose of the head and tail changes.

Indications of Imbalance in the Fascia
• Saddles are difficult to fit properly.

• Hoof- and shoe-wear patterns show quirky variations.

• The horse doesn't stand still or tie well.

• He constantly chews or mouths your lead ropes, or other objects.

• Pullbacks (on the cross-ties, for example) are common.

SOFTENING TIGHT AREAS

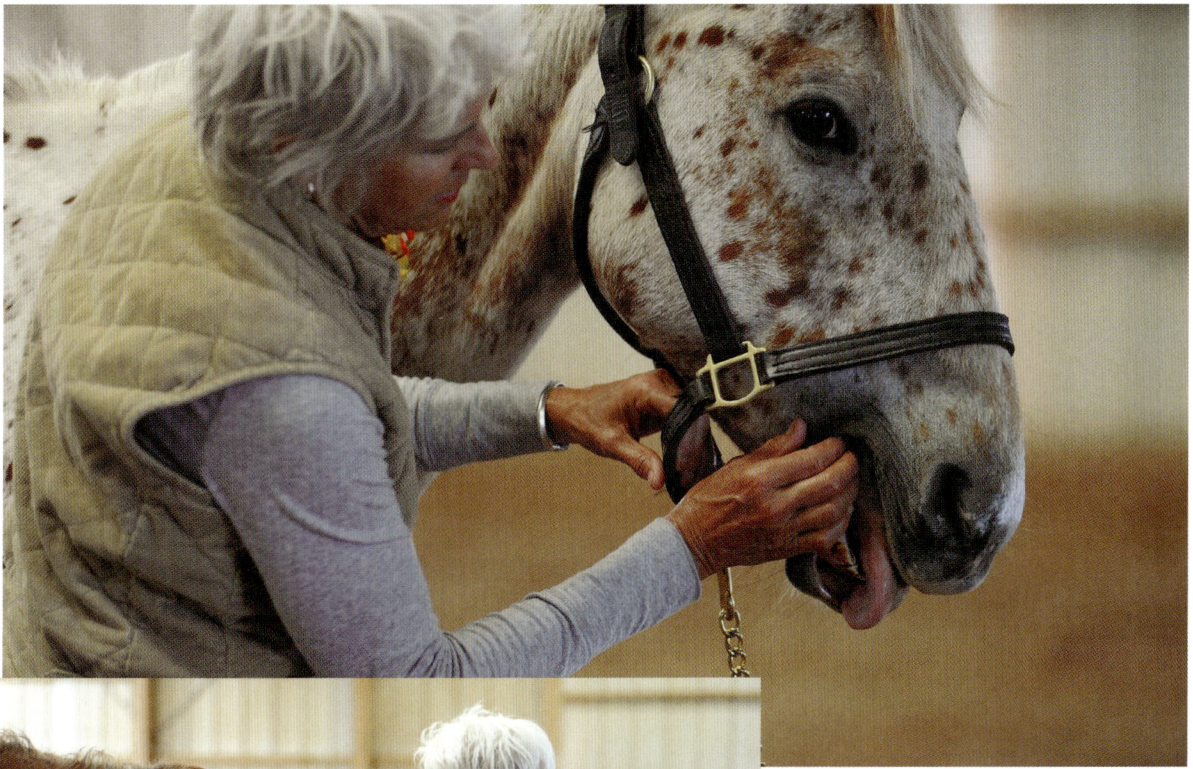

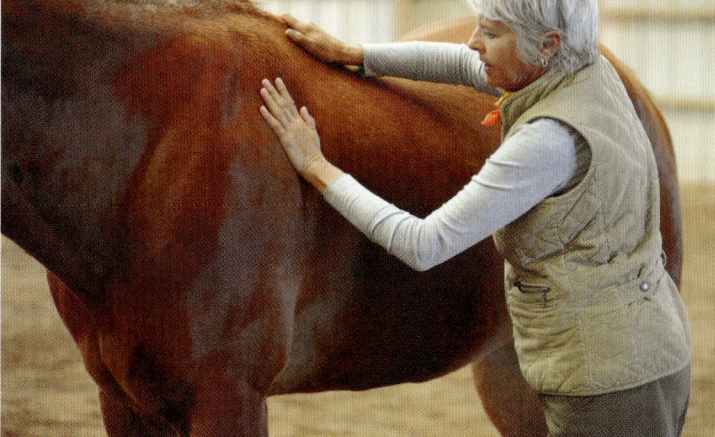

◄ **2.5** Remy, a Pony of the Americas, works his tongue as his head balances with this lower jaw change. Notice his loose lower lip. The lower lip often recedes with this head change.

▲ **2.6** This horse shows tight withers. Notice they look high when compared to the neck. Compression in the withers prevents the neck from developing. I'm using my palms here.

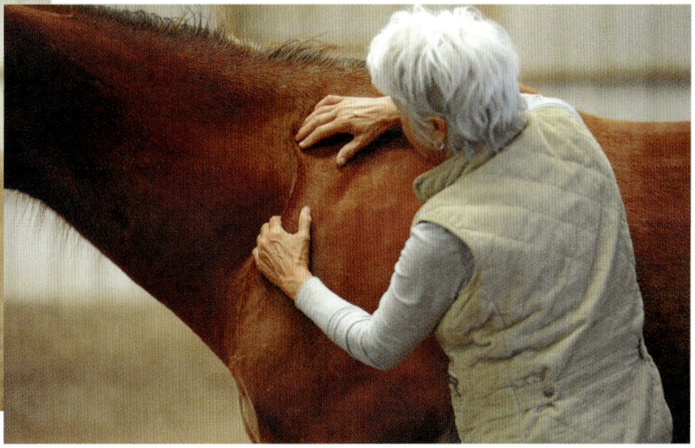

▲ **2.7** I use fingers to work the tight shoulder fascia. The upper fascia layer must be softened enough to use fingers this way. The shoulder is a key area for regular maintenance.

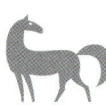

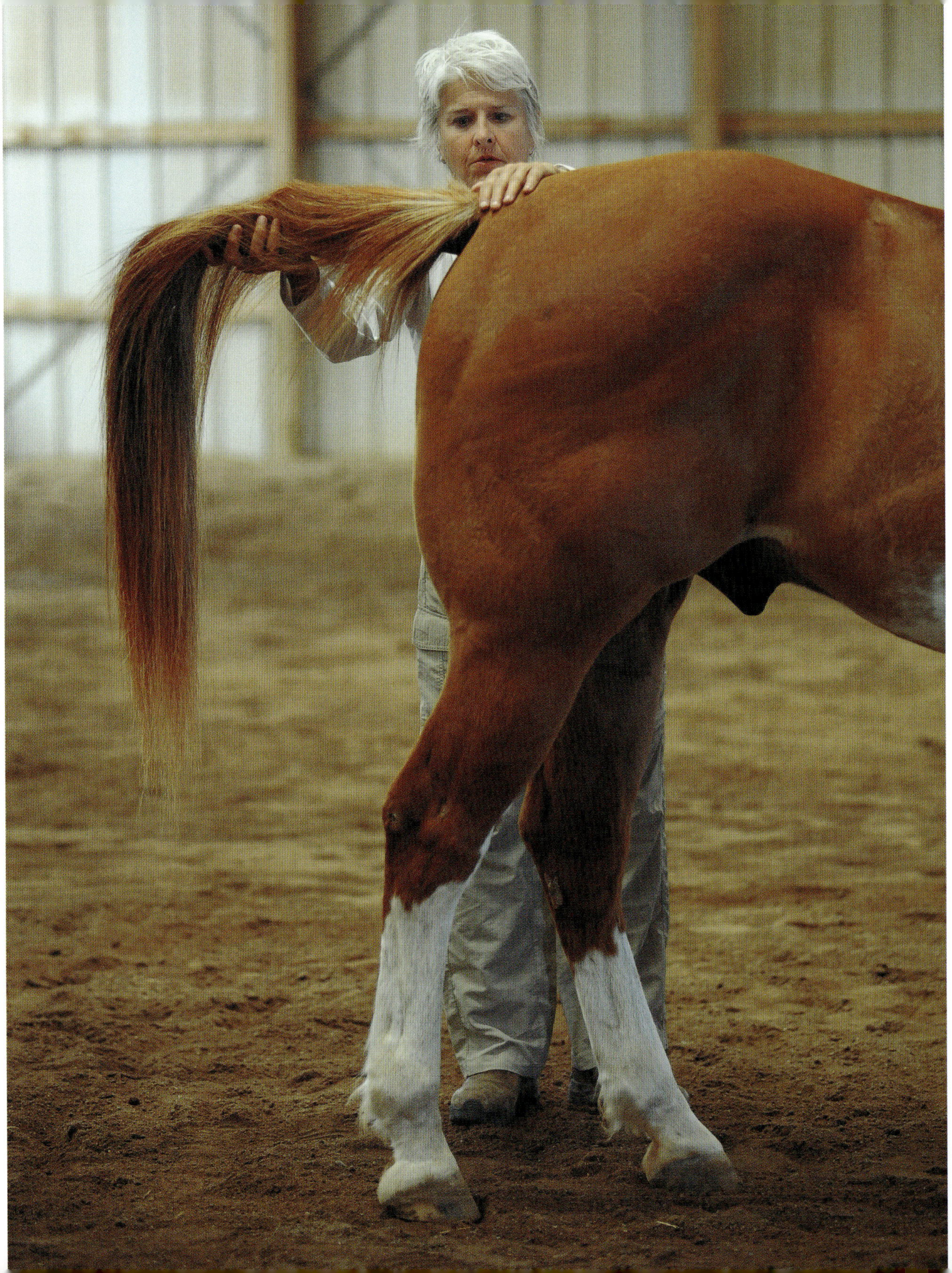

▶ **2.8** The sacral juncture is an almost numb "lost website address" for many horses. I release the dock and tail for CT, a Quarter Horse, and the sacral juncture opens much more easily.

SOFTENING TIGHT AREAS (CONTINUED)

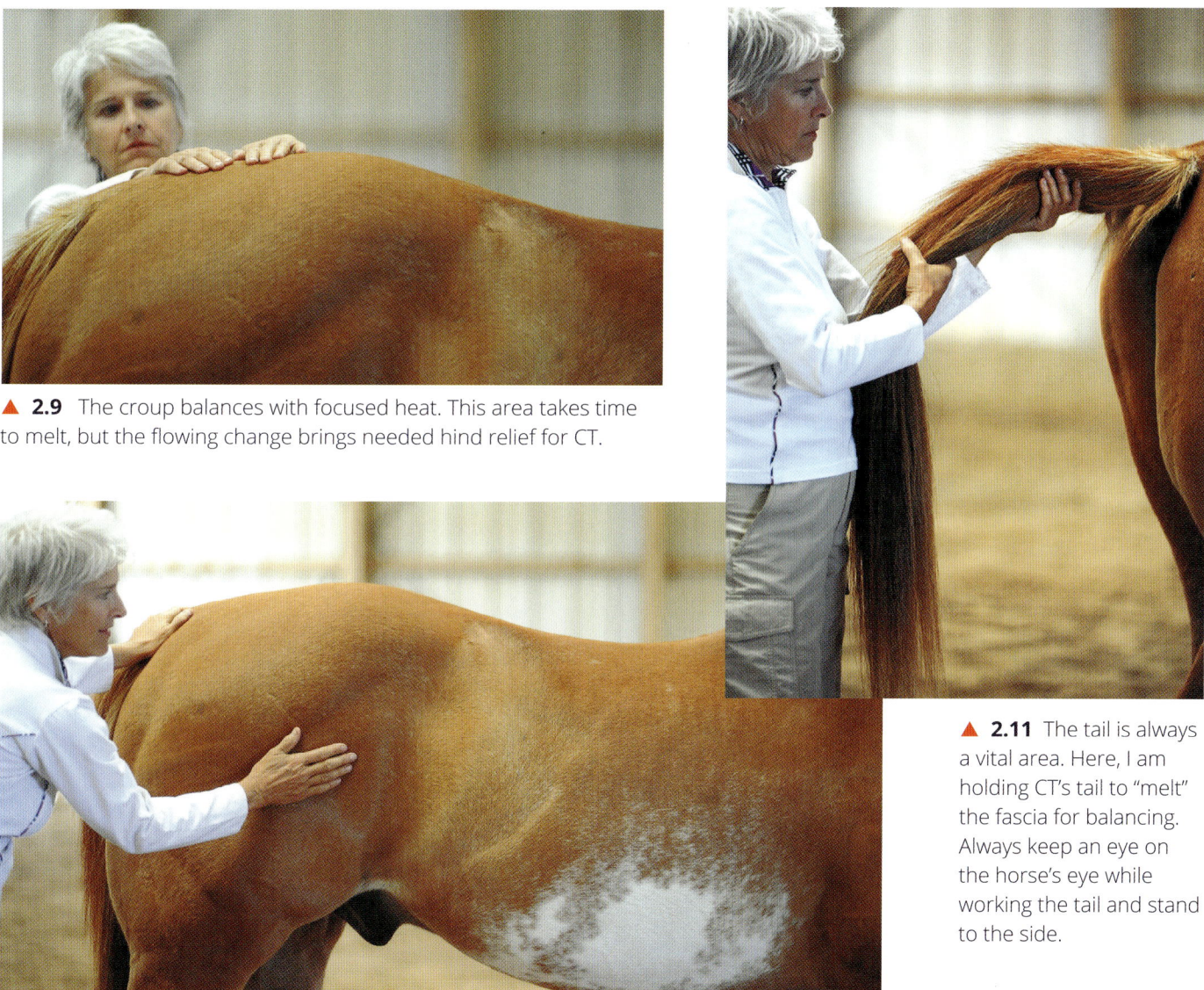

▲ **2.9** The croup balances with focused heat. This area takes time to melt, but the flowing change brings needed hind relief for CT.

▲ **2.11** The tail is always a vital area. Here, I am holding CT's tail to "melt" the fascia for balancing. Always keep an eye on the horse's eye while working the tail and stand to the side.

▲ **2.10** The area around the hip points responds well to palm work; I work wide and cup the hip points on CT with my palm.

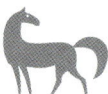

SOFTENING TIGHT AREAS (CONTINUED)

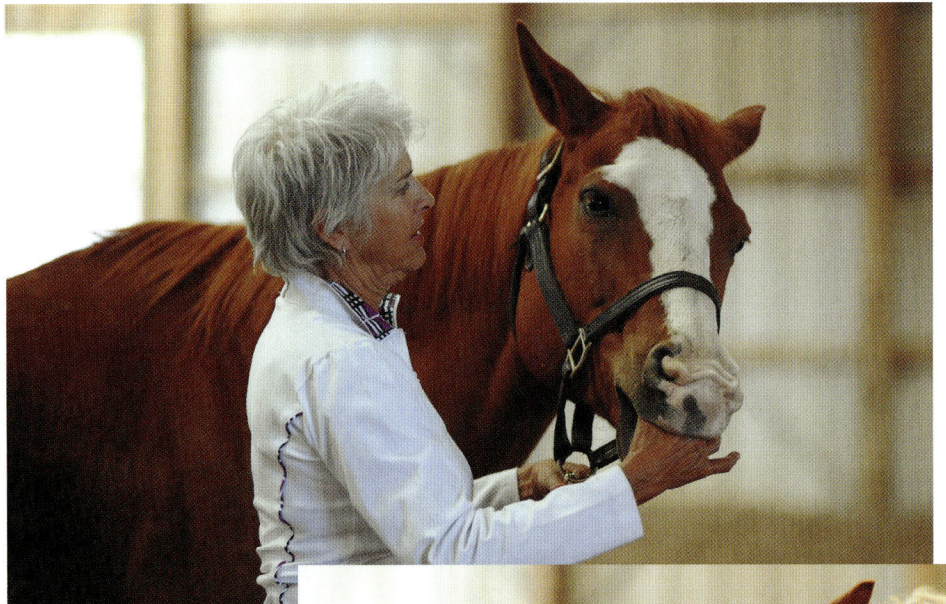

◀ **2.12** CT enjoys an in-mouth release. The dural tube, which encases the spinal cord, lengthens and brings topline change. I work the head and tail with releases to complete the "internet" connection of fascia.

▶ **2.13** Scout's tongue works as his head changes with a mouth release. My hand rests on his jaw without pressure or motion. His expression shows that he knows this is helping him.

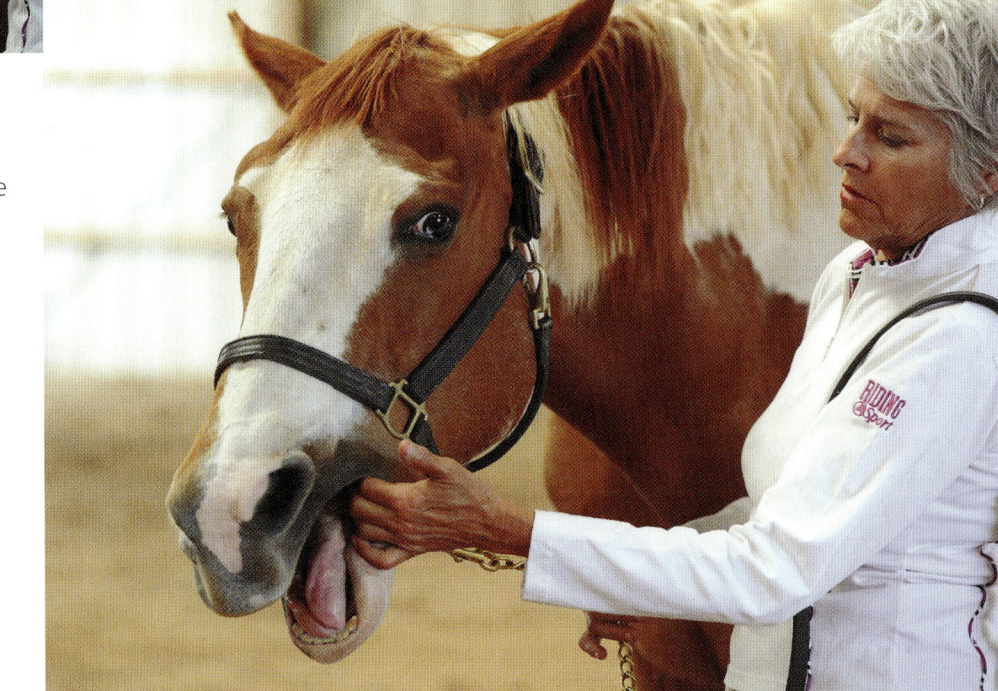

- Putting on the headstall or halter is difficult.

- He has anxious behaviors, such as spooking.

- Tacking up is difficult; the horse is often girthy.

- His tail or mane doesn't grow evenly or fully.

- His coat is dull, despite proper care and nutrition.

Using the three conformation sections as a guide for basic proportion then noticing your horse's topline carefully, you will get an overview of the tight areas, which limit fitness. In Part II, as you learn to work with the fascia changes in one area, you'll notice how other areas also change. Very tight, hard areas are the most limiting—and painful. Shoulders, withers, the sacral area, croup, and pelvis are common areas of tightness. I'm including some photos here to show you some fascia change work that deals with these tight areas (figs. 2.5–2.13).

Conformation and Self-Carriage: How Do They Connect?

As you learn to see the horse clearly, you also begin to see how conformation, which includes how he moves in real time, is connected to how he carries himself in real time. Self-carriage, or how the horse carries himself, is a conformational asset. Conformation seems to be the same as self-carriage, you might think, but self-carriage includes the horse's unique qualities of his own being.

Do you see an alert, brisk look in his eyes? Does the tail move freely when he walks? These are part of self-carriage. Self-carriage also tells you that the horse

Czar: A Hidden Glitch

Czar, an imported Warmblood, had excellent genes and was trained for jumping and dressage. Although he was young, his spine showed extreme lumbar tightness and his neck crest was eroding. Despite substantial bone and size, he didn't show enough muscle and looked underweight. He couldn't canter. His disposition was good, but he had little mental balance. These deficiencies were very unusual in his breed.

When doing a body scan on him (see how on p. 51), I found the source of trouble. His gelding scar had not healed well; many fascia compensations had grown in his groin, which inhibited his entire body's development. The slow, gentle process of melting these tight fascia-fiber adhesions took time since they had been building since he was about six months old. But the relief for Czar was immediate.

After his first session, which focused on his gelding scar release (see p. 106) and adductors, Czar stood quietly for many minutes. He seemed amazed to feel this good. In the following sessions (weekly, over three months), we balanced all the body areas that couldn't develop due to the groin fascia compression. His riding exercise was kept at the walk as he relearned his body's balance. The walk brought integration he'd never had, despite his advanced training. His conformation looked lanky at first, then progressed as muscle developed in the hind end and shoulders. The 12-session process helped the rider be able to really enjoy his education and abilities as his conformation balanced. Czar transformed from looking old at five to being the champion he truly was in eight months' time.

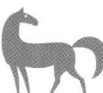

can move in an organized, healthy way with vitality, even if some topline aspects are less than completely favorable. We all know of horses that appear well built yet they lack soundness or athletic ability. Conversely, there are horses that carry themselves with talent and forward energy despite a visual flaw.

The problem of the good-looking horse that is unsound is common in the show arena and in barns. We see many new devices that improve the horse's "surface" appearance without resolving lost athletic ability. It is easy to be convinced that appearance is the whole story with a horse's conformation. Yet, appearance is only part of the horse's assets. When you include how the horse moves himself, this is where self-carriage becomes a vital aspect to true conformation.

Quick ways to simplify self-carriage are:

- Does the horse carry himself with unity, energy, and grace? Or, does he seem to be dragged around by the lead rope?

- Does he show confidence? Or is he anxious and tentative?

- Is there impulsion in his step? Free movement contrasts sharply with slow, uneven gaits.

A balanced horse is a confident horse. Self-carriage is actually not trained into the horse. It is his inborn ability to present himself and carry his muscles and other body parts efficiently and gracefully. You're putting together the puzzle on your new, expanded vision of the horse and why he looks, moves, and acts as he does. Without balanced conformation, self-carriage will lack unity, grace, and impulsion. The horse will also lack the sparkle of vitality. Both balanced conformation and vibrant self-carriage depend on fit, healthy, fascial connections throughout the horse's body.

> Self-carriage is a means for the horse to express his unique talent of being himself. It shows us immediately how comfortable the horse is with himself.

Record a Conformation Inventory

Many riders see their horses daily or several times weekly so changes are hard to recall. What you notice with delight or concern one day fades quickly in the stream of days. It's hard to keep track of what's wrong, as well as what's right with your horse.

Digital photos are extremely useful for conformation assessment (figs. 2.14–2.18). The habit of using photos trains your eyes. A photo of the four views shows you how your horse is progressing (even professionals forget how much a horse can change). I use quick photos taken on a tablet or an easy camera to record the horse's change objectively. The photos are even dated for convenience. Somehow, changes jump out faster to the eye when you look at the horse on a screen. If you are not computer-oriented, you can take photos and print them. Even sketches will help you to track what's happening with your horse.

The photo is especially useful with key changes like the muzzle, stance, and topline. In fact, the topline is much easier to assess in a photo. These records support your time investment and bring a true feeling of empowerment for helping your horse.

CONFORMATION INVENTORY

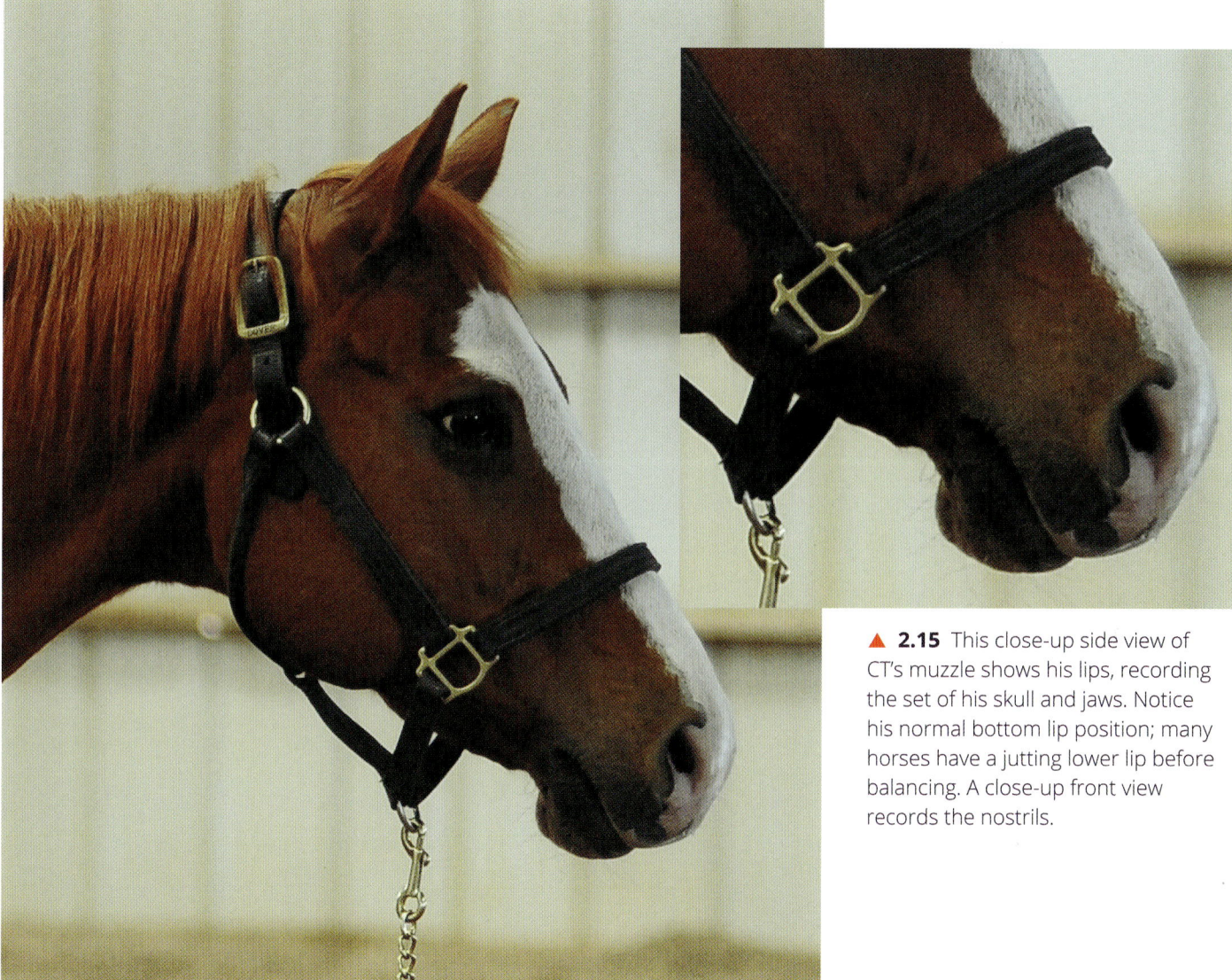

▲ **2.15** This close-up side view of CT's muzzle shows his lips, recording the set of his skull and jaws. Notice his normal bottom lip position; many horses have a jutting lower lip before balancing. A close-up front view records the nostrils.

▲ **2.14** CT is our model for the head view digital record. A close-up of the head focuses our attention on the profile details. This side view is a basic record to take before starting changes.

CONFORMATION INVENTORY (CONTINUED)

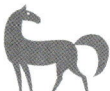

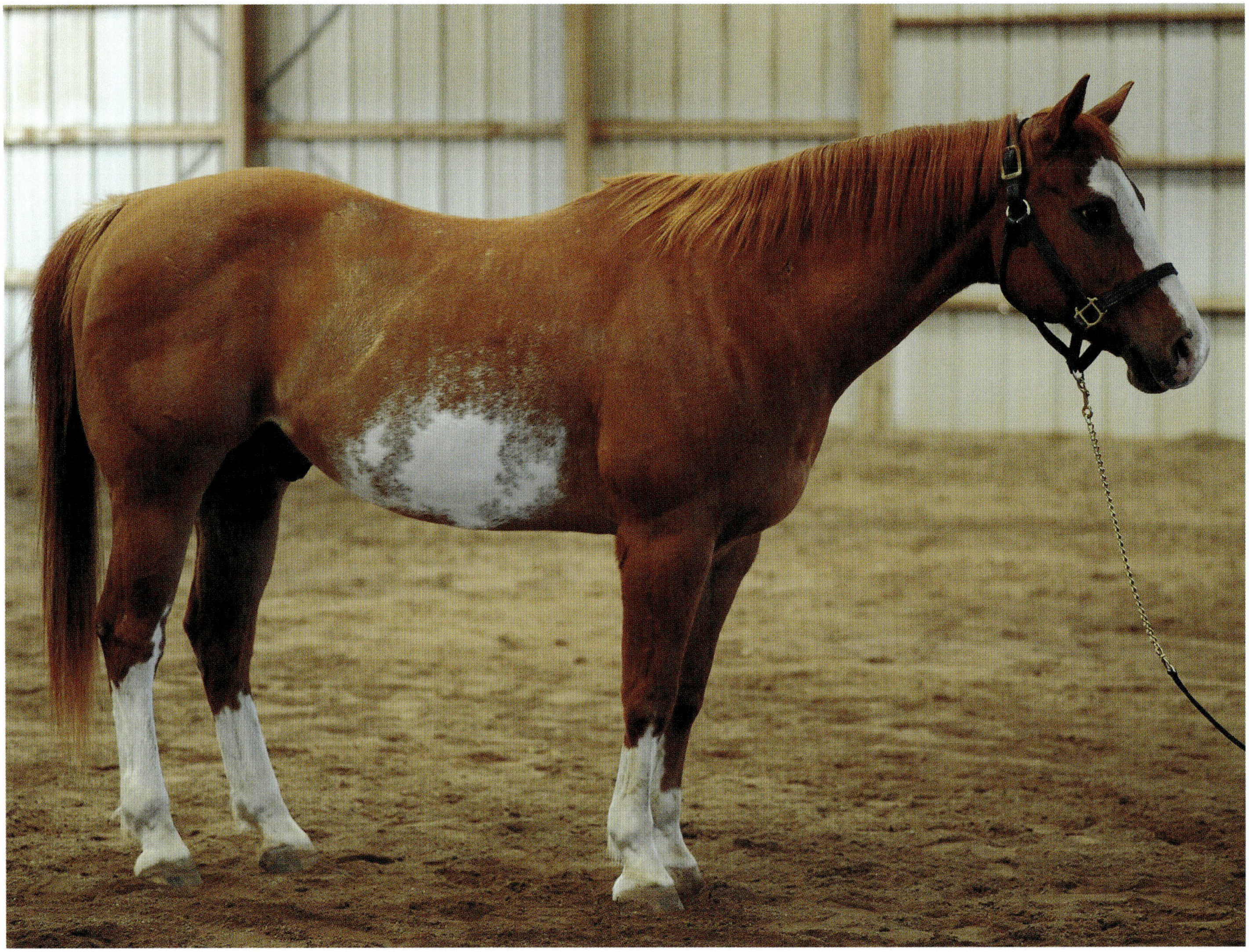

▲ **2.16** A full view of the horse, however he stands, is a vital record. We photograph both sides, in case there are differences. CT shows a balanced front stance with a slightly offset rear stance.

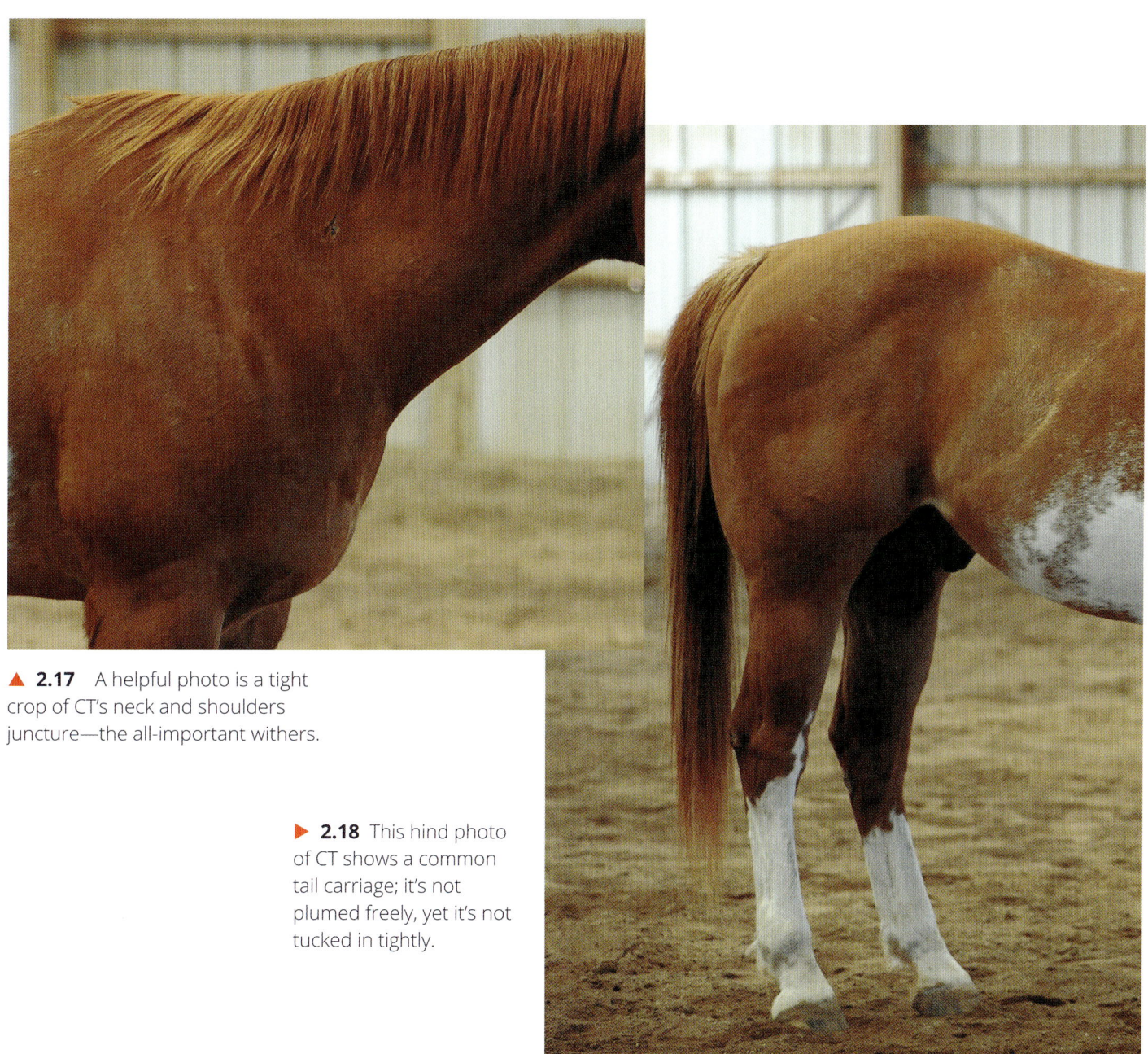

▲ **2.17** A helpful photo is a tight crop of CT's neck and shoulders juncture—the all-important withers.

▶ **2.18** This hind photo of CT shows a common tail carriage; it's not plumed freely, yet it's not tucked in tightly.

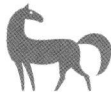

Four Views to Record

1. Digital photos of both sides, front, and rear.

2. Head photos, front and both sides.

3. Close-up of muzzle's side view and front view, including nostrils.

4. Stance photos; both sides; from about 8 yards.

Photo Inventory Tips

- Position the horse against a neutral background. Avoid visual distractions that confuse the eye, like barrels or poles.

- If possible, use the same photographic background each time. This information is very energizing and creates powerful incentive to improve your horse with this work, as well as appreciating his progress. The horse changes dramatically in a year, so your files will be invaluable.

- Print out the photos, whether at home or with a commercial printer; you keep these large prints for reference and progress checks. The photos are extremely useful in defeating the critic, whether inner or outer. We'll be discussing this critic more in chapter 8 (see p. 128).

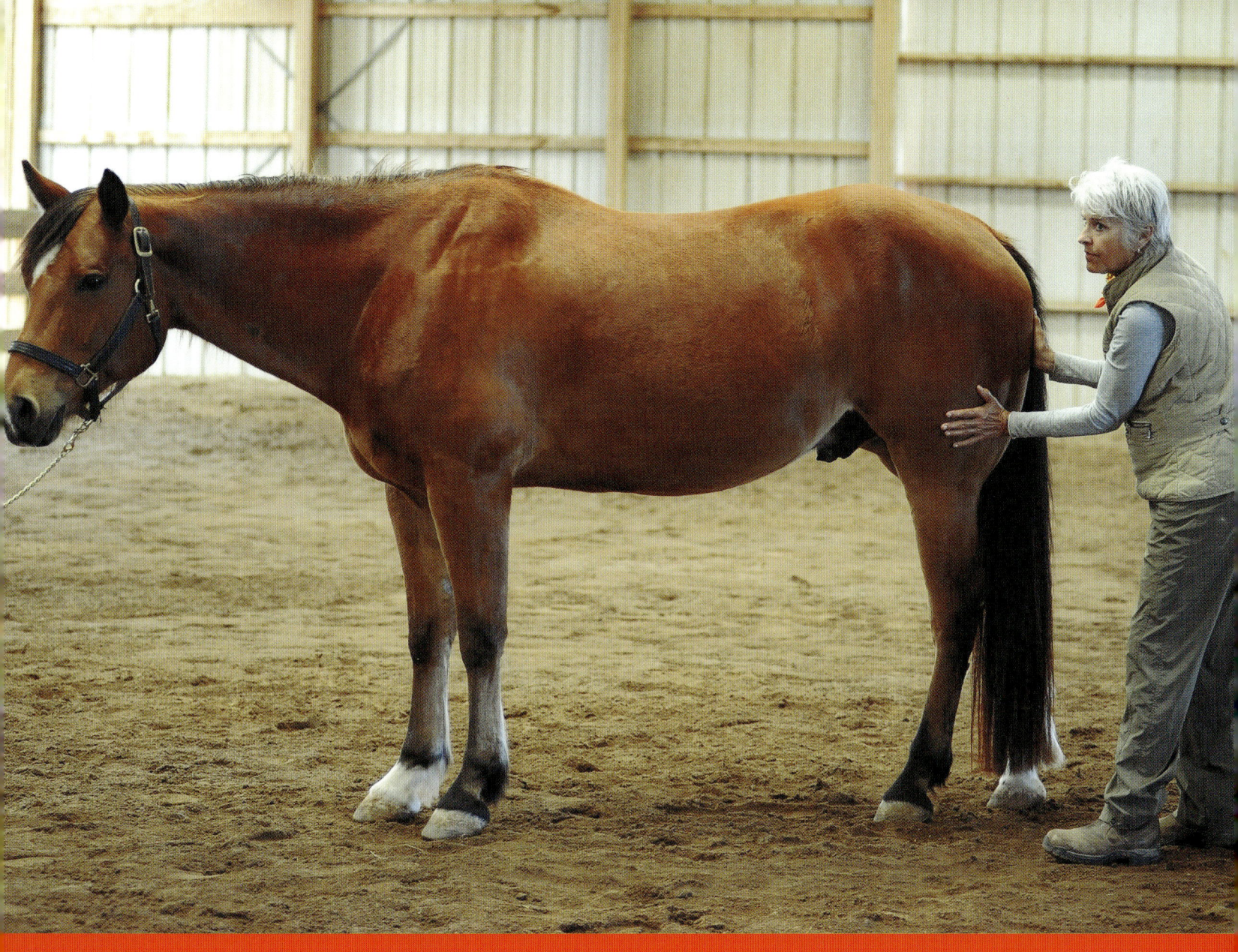

3 | A Balanced Stance

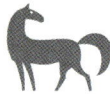

Red: A Long Struggle

Red was an example of a horse well equipped to do his job as a family trail horse following a career as a lesson horse for hunter jumpers. But his natural conformation was altered by human "improvements" when his normal front foot was trimmed to match his clubfoot. An unsound horse is a horse in trouble.

Red's story is typical in the horse world, although the clubfoot is found in only a small percentage of horses. As an experienced, wise farrier commented, "He knows how to move and use his body. When his feet are trimmed to match evenly, it throws him off. He was born with a size one foot on the left and a size two foot on the right." The attempt to even his front hooves brought lameness blocking his entire life path. Hiding a body problem leaves the horse stuck with even more compensation.

Recurring lameness was the initial main complaint of a new owner. He had no trot, from a walk he galloped; hills caused him anxiety. His feet were shod with all four in matching shoes when she purchased Red. Three months later, his front feet looked very odd. The left foot was a size one shoe, round and smaller, while the right one was a larger size two, oval. Red's pleasant and sincere personality kept the owner riding him and trying to discover what the missing pieces were. The farrier confirmed the truth that his front feet were different sizes and the left foot was a clubfoot. His hindquarters were very undeveloped for his size. Also, his withers were very high and paired with a ewe neck, despite good breeding.

As the front feet grew to their normal size and shape, a left shoulder emerged as Red's core problem; it compensated for his clubfoot. His feet may have been trimmed to match for many years forcing him to continually struggle with his center of gravity, the shoulders. With his shoulders compromised, Red's hindquarters couldn't develop properly. The shoulder imbalance also compressed his withers and neck, preventing length and cresting.

For Red, five months of regular bodywork and gentle riding at the walk brought soundness and confidence. His shoulder creases opened fully after six weeks, which stabilized his center of gravity. Hindquarters balance allowed his loins to tuck for rear traction and he came off the forehand. His cribbing habit disappeared with the cranial and poll changes. A natural foot size ended knee compensations, which had caused his stumbling. He resumed a useful life as a sound and pleasant trail mount for his family, a job he loved.

Stance Supports the Topline

As I noted in the last chapter, the line along the "horizon" of the horse's body from nose to tail tip, the topline, responds quickly to fascia changes. You watch the topline for the first clues to major changes taking place in a horse's conformation. Using photos, you will see topline changes in as little as a one-hour session. Poll changes quickly improve cresting, while neck balancing lengthens the neck. As always, it takes what it takes, but you're now on the path of progress for your horse.

The three body sections (see p. 26), however, take longer to balance when one is larger than the other two; the horse has a large body and one section may weigh 450 pounds. This is why the topline changes show up earlier. Underneath the topline and the body, the horse's legs are the supports.

The horse's stance is how he stands when he's at ease. Here you see where he places his feet, if he stands straight laterally as well as front to back, and how his neck holds his head. The "box" is used to describe a horse that is standing square and has each leg directly under him, like the legs of a table. This is the most balanced standing position for a horse.

The horse's stance tells you right away how balanced he is. Any hindquarters imbalance or restriction shows in the stance position, as well as shoulder imbalances. Stance also shows lateral imbalance, which is when the front or hind legs don't line up. Stance variations show up well in your photo record inventory so if you don't notice them when just looking at your horse, you will certainly notice these variations in the photos.

As you know, many horses do not stand "in the box" often. A common conformation reason for this is that

> ## VARIATIONS IN STANCE
>
> - Feet don't make a "box" shape.
> - Tripod: two feet are very close together, creating a "tripod" look.
> - Splayed feet.
> - Toes-out or toes-in.
> - Stretched out: legs aren't under the shoulders or the pelvis.
> - Offset (usually the hind feet).

the sacral and pelvic area has tight fascia adhesions pulling his hind legs into an offset stance. He can't stand straight easily, because his tissue is twisted and tight. Fascia balancing in the hindquarters and shoulders advances the horse's stance. Head balancing helps him to maintain the gains. The hind end won't retain balance unless the head is also balanced. The head and hind are the two balance points for self-carriage, mentioned in the last chapter.

Offset Stance

Stance is an excellent quick guide for checking for strain of any kind in the horse. With strain, or even mild injury, the horse usually doesn't stand square. The usual stance of the horse shows how balanced he is (fig. 3.1). Many of us have seen horses stand in awkward positions. Often,

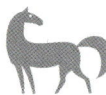

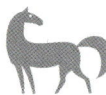

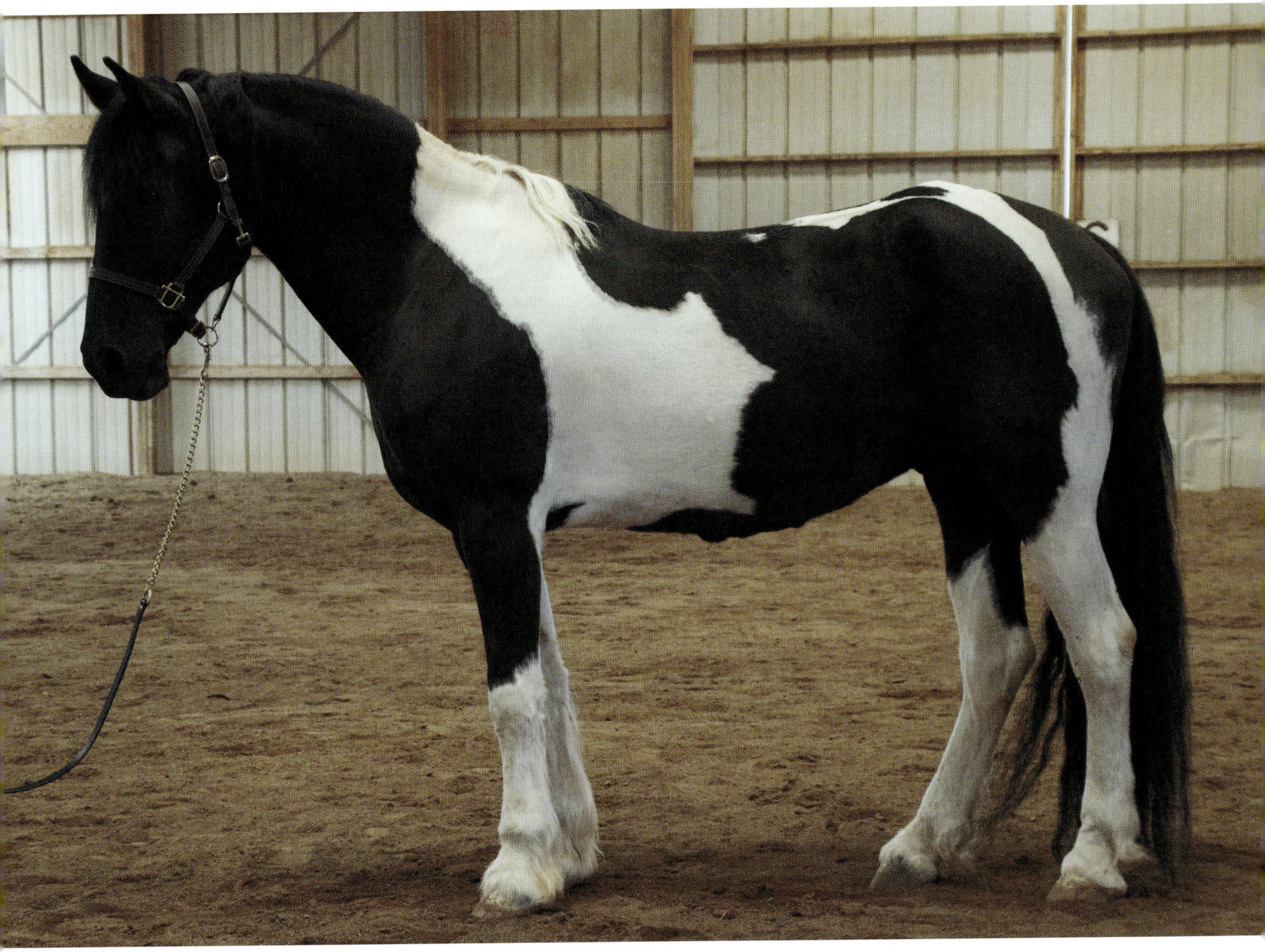

▲ **3.1** This shows Beau's stance and topline. Notice his hind legs are offset, indicating imbalance. His back shows less than the usual desired muscle. His thick tail is free and loose, but not plumed.

we notice this, but don't give it much thought. An awkward stance shows a completely dysfunctional balance in a running animal, and stance is a quick clue to pelvic imbalance and shoulder problems.

A balanced horse goes easily into a "box" stance often. He does not cross his legs awkwardly or stand on top of his own feet, as I have seen some horses do. Offset hind-leg positions of any kind always indicate deep fascial strains that limit canter leads, collection, and even walking straight. Often, these are not difficult imbalances to release.

This offset stance is not about cosmetic appearances. You should always look at hind-leg stance when assessing conformation and movement of the horse. If the horse doesn't look balanced and in even proportion, he usually doesn't move consistently well. Sometimes, it takes about 10 minutes to watch the horse as he stands. Some horses come to balance quickly, while others move around or stand at rest before coming to their own usual stance. Also, you'll notice the front leg to hind leg relationship.

With practice, you will learn to notice if the spacing is even or where it varies. An example of spacing is when the front hooves are wider spaced than the hind hooves. Or, in reverse, the hind hooves are wider than the front. Look for each leg to be square under that corner of the body, like the table I mentioned earlier.

A reminder here, an offset stance does not imply lack of genetic gifts, it's a fascia-balancing situation. In fact, while the hind legs can look very awkward on a horse, they usually respond very quickly to balancing. Common examples of these advances include the

> Stance becomes your best quick guide to keeping track of your horse's balance.

"tripod" stance where the front legs look balanced but the hind legs are very close together, with one hoof usually farther forward than the other. This stance is very common for horses with hindquarters or pelvic imbalance.

However, great news: it's usually quite simple to progress to a balanced stance with regular fascia changes. No matter how unbalanced your horse is, steady contact with sensitive hands leads you quickly to find the fascial problems. Continual progress photos show you how your horse's conformation is realigning under your touch. Over a few months of steady contact, the topline and stance organize for balance and your horse's mental poise will dramatically improve as he feels safer.

Head and Neck

After you notice how the horse stands, you can look at his head and neck. The neck's length, curve, and shape tells you how balanced the front of the horse is. Most often, a thin, undeveloped neck means that the shoulders are extremely tight, preventing the neck from developing. The poll won't have flexion on a tight neck. So, in an overall view of the front, the neck's situation points you to the need for head and poll balancing, as well as major fascia release work in the shoulders, shoulder creases, and withers.

A tight poll, tight jaws, and tight head fascia also result in an inability of the horse to breathe easily. This is often the source of panic attacks. While the phrase "may limit the horse's breathing" sounds relatively benign, let's consider how a human athlete would react

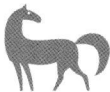

to obstructed breathing while performing his high-level sport. Lack of oxygen is not an asset while attempting complex athletic movement of any kind. Worst of all, cells are dying without oxygen.

As you work with the horse's head, neck, poll, and shoulders, the fascia is restructuring. There is more space between the parts. Often, the horse gets a loose and lean look, with some areas looking bony and not muscled. This bony look particularly occurs in the withers and shoulders. You don't need to worry about these in-between phases. These changes all balance themselves as the fascia changes continue.

This is another reason why although a little fascial balancing helps, a little won't bring you a great looking horse instantly. Like a house, you have to finish the building process. While you can pace the sessions according to your choice, it's good to keep the process ongoing—even with short sessions—for the best results in the fascial internet. The tight fascia must balance enough to allow muscles and groups of muscles to develop fully.

Shoulders and Hindquarters

When you work with hindquarters' fascia to improve stance, the muscles develop better tone and shape. Light hind ends become substantial. As you open tight shoulder fascia, muscle builds to fill in hollows in the withers and shoulders. Shoulder-crease openings, which you'll learn about in chapter 5 (see p. 91), will allow the neck to lengthen and muscle to build on the crest and poll. All the new space you create, as the tight fascia opens, allows the muscles to develop and the body to balance. This is how the horse's shape improves so dramatically.

Gaunt, tight horses fill out with muscle, while paunchy horses gain an athletic, trim body.

Progress Changes to Watch For
- The three sections of the horse's conformation become more equal.
- Dips and lumps in the topline disappear.
- The horse stands more in the box.
- Head carriage is balanced, not low or high.
- The poll elevates and flexes into a more collected look.
- Tail carriage becomes plumed and expressive.

Tail

I've mentioned how the tail fits into the topline assessment. We've also discussed how the tail demonstrates vitality in self-carriage. Let's clarify more details regarding the tail since it is so important to the balance of the hindquarters of the horse. The short list below details the most common tail problems. A rigid, clamped tail is found in about 35 percent of horses. While it seems a cosmetic issue, tail flexibility is a big deal regarding hindquarters power and flexion.

When you look at the horse's stance, also notice how his tail hangs. The tail position shows you a lot about his pelvic balance. You can save yourself much time restoring the hindquarters balance by handling the tail to release rigidity for complete flexion. Tail changes efficiently help resolve hind imbalances in an off stance of any kind.

I discuss the tail in more detail in chapters 4 and 5.

Tail Variations Indicating Back Tension and Pelvic Strain

- A clamped tail, pressing into the hindquarters.

- Tail that pulls more to one side.

- Tail is twisted, has knobs, or is very rigid.

Now, you've learned how to assess the horse's conformation and stance. You also know how to see his three sections: nose to withers; barrel, hindquarters. You see his horizon line—the topline—clearly. And, you know the four supporting legs show how balanced his stance is. You've practiced recording his present assets with photos. You understand that his stance reveals his fascia's imbalance, which affects how well he can move under saddle.

Photos show the truth of these three main aspects of conformational balance, and also show areas to progress for the horse. You are beginning to see how he fits together now and you know how he feels under saddle. This sharper vision of your horse, coupled with your riding experience, brings motivation to advance your horse so he can do more and feel better.

By now, the dots are connecting for how the horse's fascial internet controls work, how his conformation, his topline, and how he stands affect him. If you love progress, you are impatient to get busy and find out exactly what his blockages are. But before you touch the horse and feel the fascia, let's go over safety when handling horses, whether your own or someone else's.

When the horse has had all the fascia changes he wants, he "flicks" you away. This way, there is never too much change.

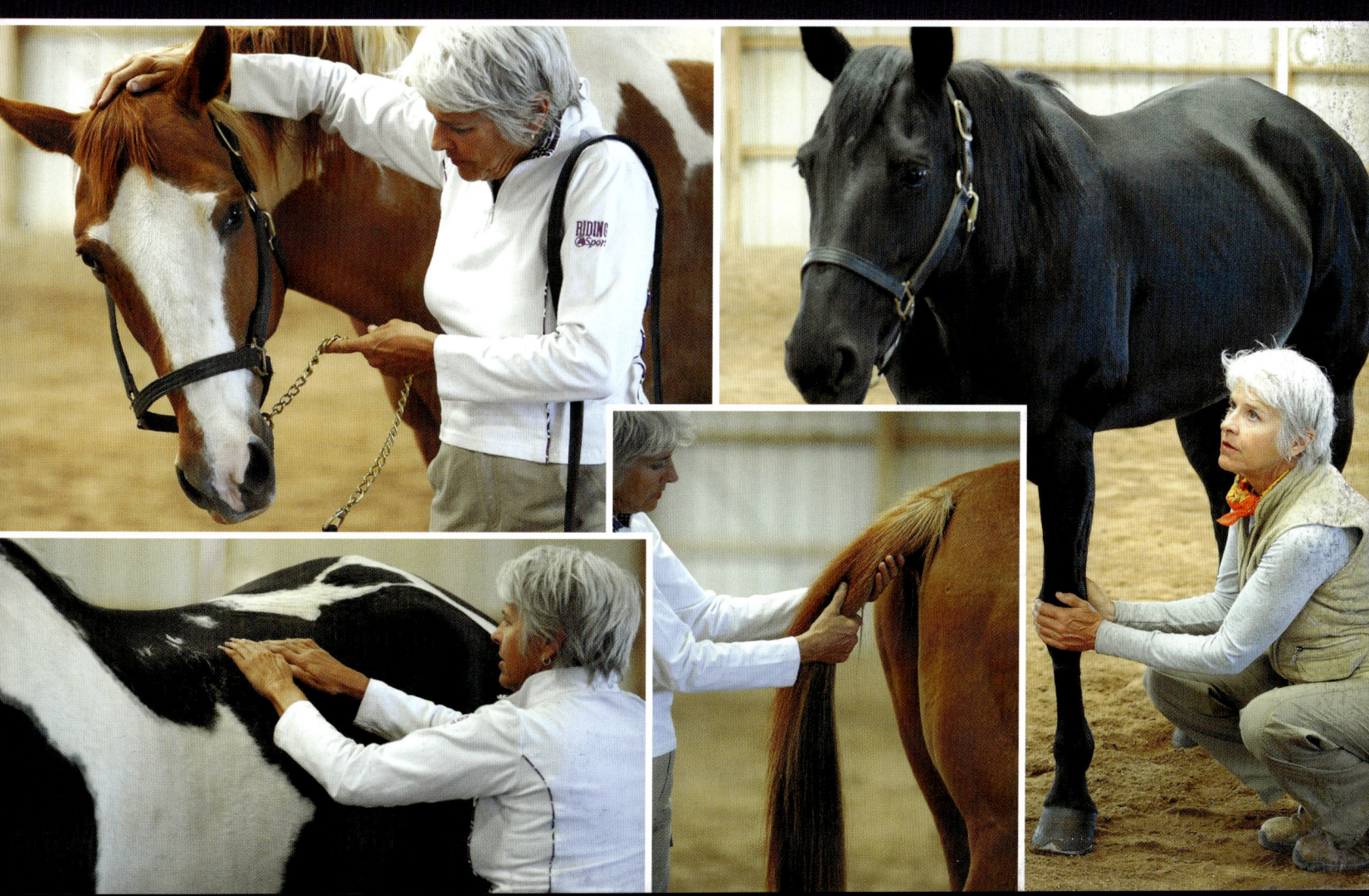

PART II

Conformation Balancing:
The Fascia-Change Work

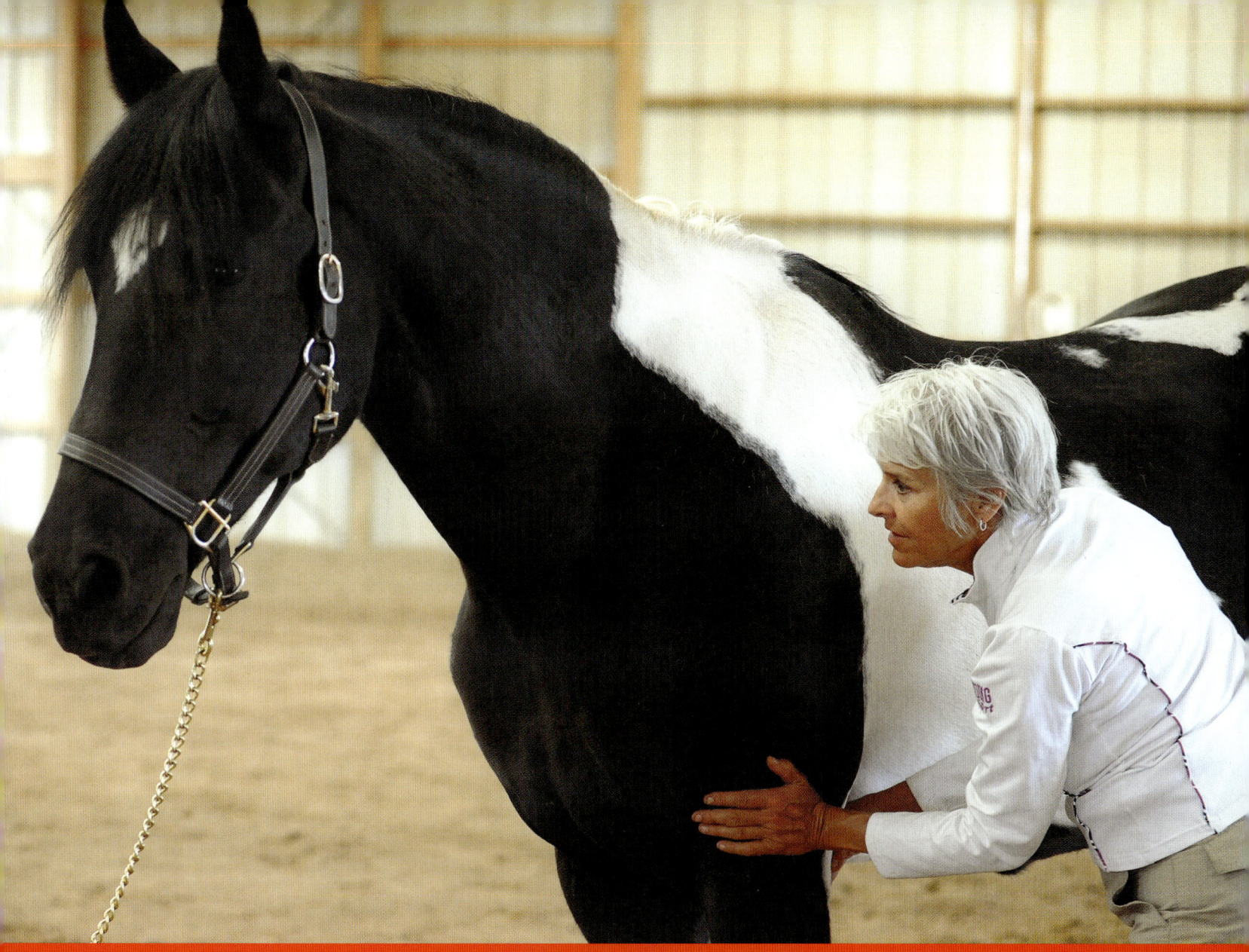

4 | Your Hands on the Horse

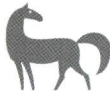

Safety in Bodywork

Before you begin, it is important to consider some general safety rules and work manners:

- The Number One Rule: Only work with the horse's full agreement.
- Always be aware of the horse's power and ability to move instantly.
- Safety is first priority at all times.

Joe: A Cowboy Hat Incident

While doing a session alone in a well-maintained barn with wide aisles, I worked with a calm, older Thoroughbred named Joe. At the owner's direction, Joe was tied to a rebar pole in the stall door (using a quick-release knot). The air was still. I was working at the hind end, standing to the side of the horse as I teach my students to do, when a sudden gust of wind lifted a white straw cowboy hat off its hook and carried it six feet in the air. As the white hat sailed past us both, the startled horse pulled back and sank on his haunches. I easily stepped farther from him. Joe bent the rebar, although the quick release knot held. The hat slid to the ground when the gust left.

This is a good example of a time I was very glad to be standing at the side rather than behind the horse!

- Never insist on meeting a goal.
- Prevent commotion: machines, dogs, and interruptions included.
- Pay attention to the horse's eyes and ears for his approval.
- Work in a large area; choose paddocks, corrals and wash-rack areas.
- Do not stand between the horse and a wall or fence.
- Keep your feet directly under your shoulders.
- Stand to the side of the horse; be able to step away.
- Avoid putting your head over parts of the horse's body, especially his head.
- Be aware of weather conditions: wind, storms, and air pressure affect horses.
- Your headgear should always allow peripheral vision.
- Allow the horse to move and turn if he chooses; it helps the release.
- Verbally encourage the horse to support his feeling of change; be present for him.
- Come to the horse with a quiet, open, and peaceful mind—not anger or tension.
- Never hurry work.
- An interruption during a stroke or release should be avoided—it insults the horse.
- Check jewelry for sharp edges or, better still, remove any.

- Chemical odors are off putting; consider using only mild castile soap.

- Wash hands before working—and between working different horses.

- Use eye protection when handling the tail. Hair whip-lash is painful.

- Working at scheduled feeding times is not advised; meals are priority for horses.

- Bodywork should wait until fresh wounds, skin conditions, or diseases are healed completely. When there is illness in the barn, wait until the crisis is over.

Guarding

I use the word "guarding" for horses that respond aggressively to contact, or might do so. A non-judgmental approach helps you remember that the horse's main concern is being protected from insensitive handling or intolerable contact. Judgment creates tension during bodywork and the horse feels this immediately (see p. 140 for telepathy).

Patience and acceptance bring the best results. When a horse is guarding, only use contact that he will accept and do not consider this a loss of authority on your part. Advancement in contact results from *trust*. Watch for "approval cues" that indicate fascia changes, keeping an eye on his eye and ears.

Irritation Warning Cues
- Ears go back or flatten.

- Tail-swishing.

- Feet-stomping or moving.

- Head-turning or swiping.

- Tension in body.

- Back-arching.

- Eye showing anxiety.

Approval Cues
- Gurgling sounds in the guts or stomach.

- "Still Point" inner gazes.

- Licking and chewing.

- Muzzle-twitching.

- Eye-blinking and staring.

- Hind-leg flexing.

- Yawning, snorting, sighing.

- Stretching out.

- Head-dropping.

- Leaning into the contact.

- Lips quivering.

The Body Scan

Your Conformation Balancing hands-on work starts with the body scan. In the scan, you examine the horse's body using a flowing motion with your hands, from neck to hind. This fluid motion of feeling the horse's body begins your session with the horse.

The body scan identifies sensitive areas, acquaints you with the horse's condition, and informs the horse

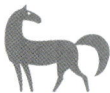

HOW TO SCAN:
A Photo Reference Guide

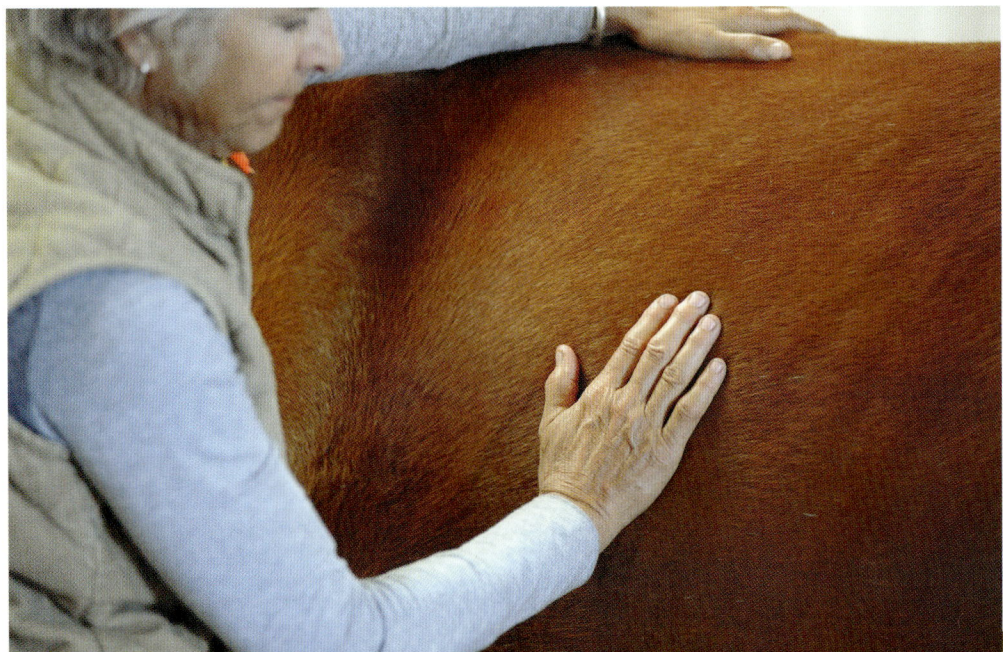

◀ **4.1** A palm is highly effective in all sensitive areas and delivers the most heat to adhesions. While it may look too easy, a palm is profoundly effective. Here, I feel the ribs, often a very sensitive area for horses.

▶ **4.2** A palm easily creates a smoothing flow for the horse, which is very relaxing and allows him to sink into his sensations while enabling me to feel the horse's structure.

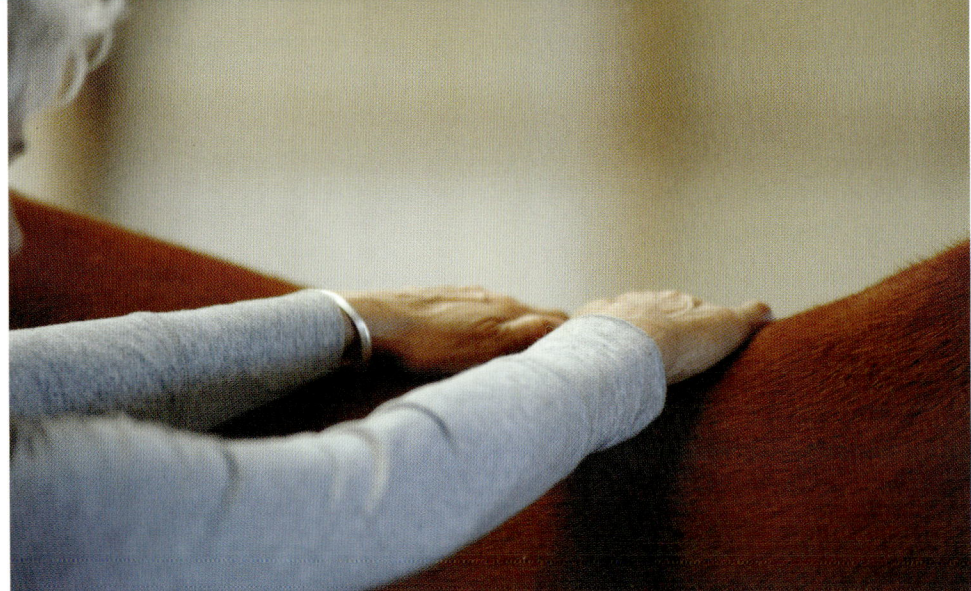

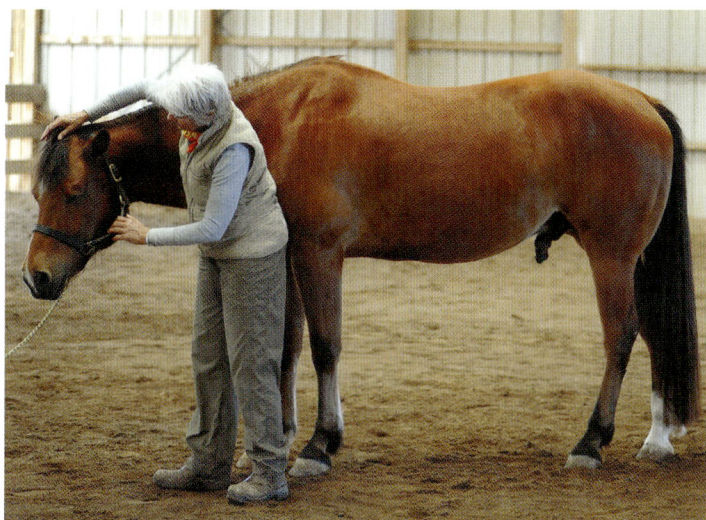

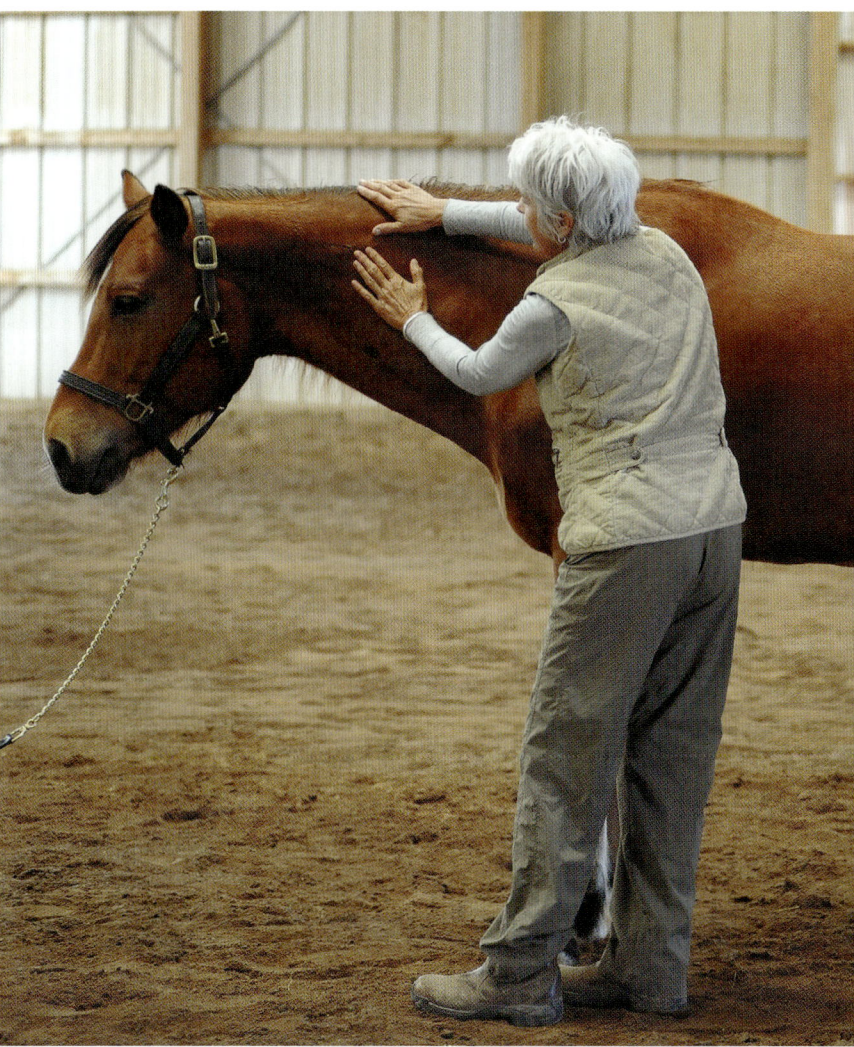

◄ 4.3 "EZ," a Quarter Horse, is the model for the scan. I use a palm to feel the fascia under the skin. A scan can start anywhere on the horse; but I don't choose difficult areas. EZ is relaxed and attentive.

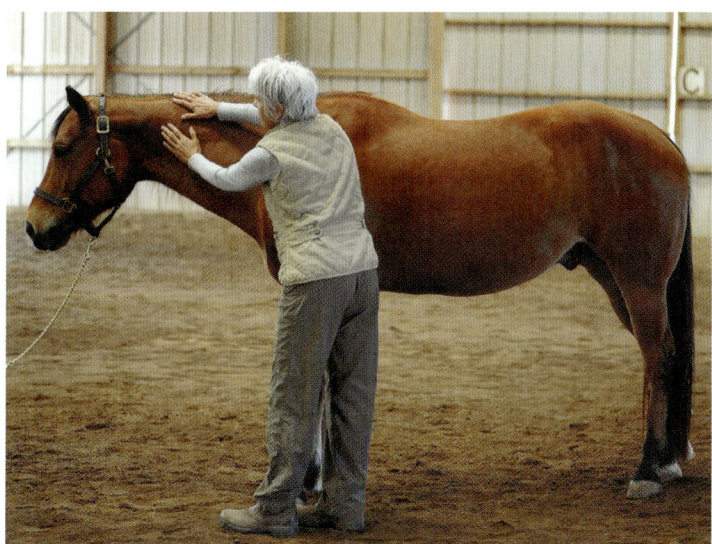

▲ 4.4 EZ enjoys feeling my contact as my palms flow over his neck. The horse learns in the scan that this contact doesn't hurt or irritate him. The contact flows without jerks or interruption.

▲ 4.5 I sweep EZ's neck in the direction of the hair.

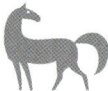

HOW TO SCAN (CONTINUED)

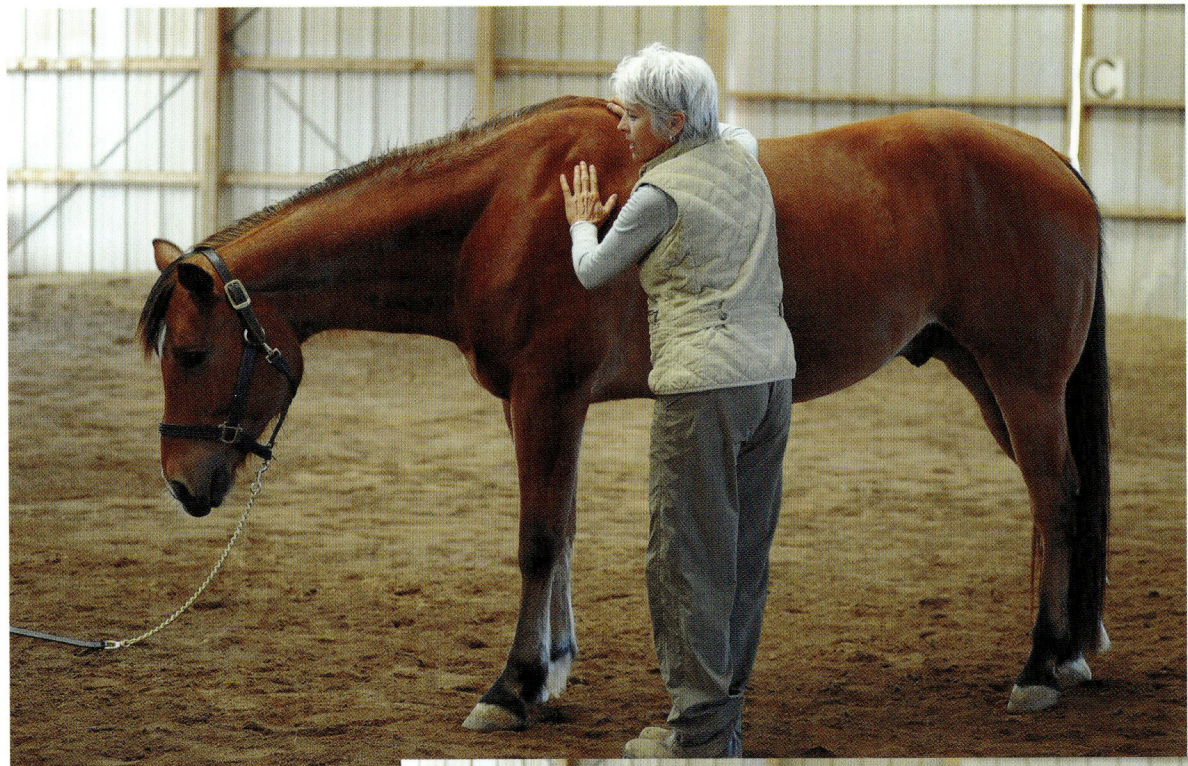

◀ **4.6** The shoulder scan relaxes EZ and his head drops. I cover the entire horse, both sides, in the scan.

▶ **4.7** Sensitive areas, such as the barrel, are treated with care in the scan; EZ is very relaxed.

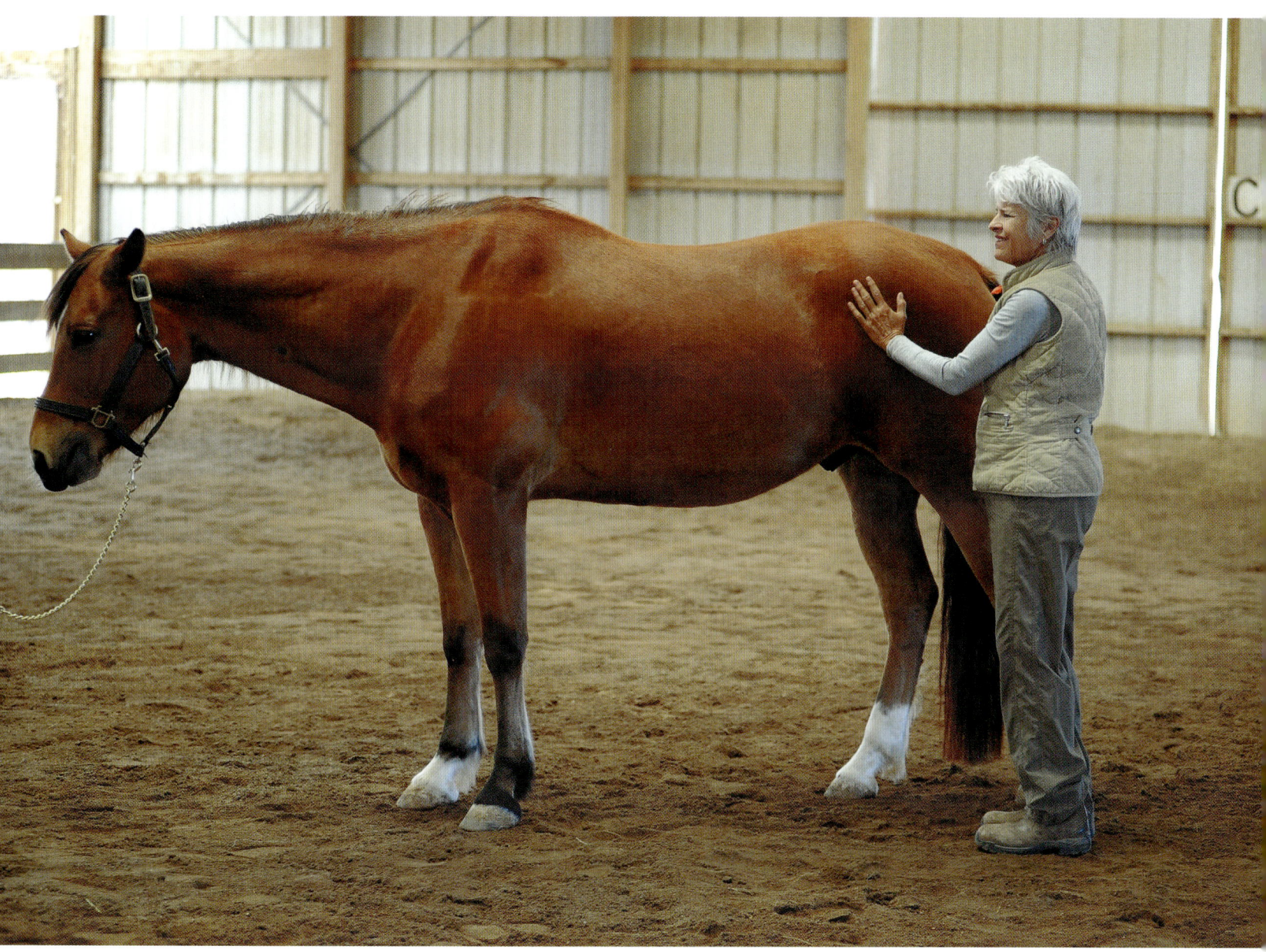

▲ **4.8** The hip is scanned, still using the palm.

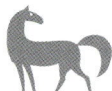

HOW TO SCAN (CONTINUED)

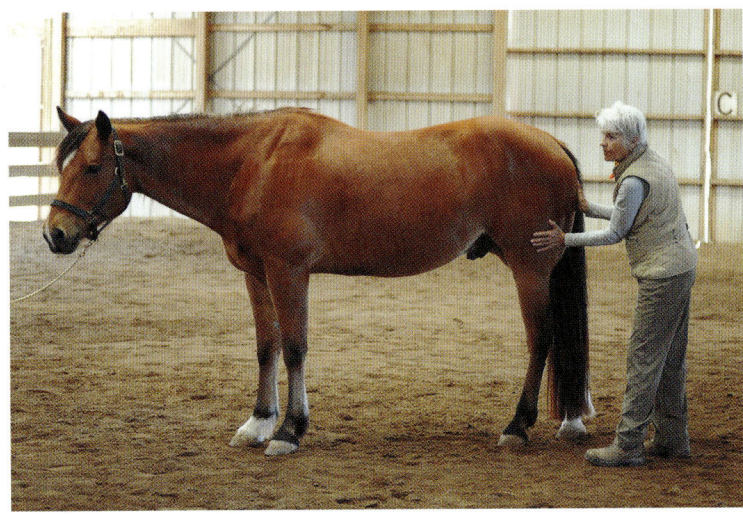

▲ **4.9** Hindquarters are often sensitive; watch for guarding.

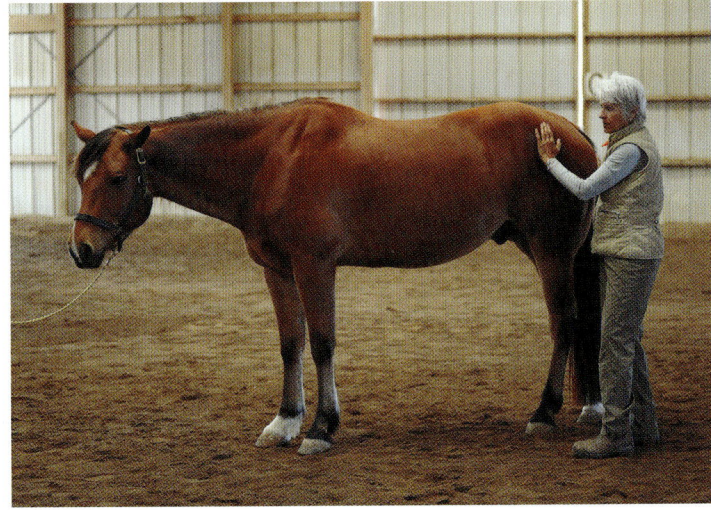

▲ **4.10** EZ is not sensitive in his flank; always stand to the side of the horse here.

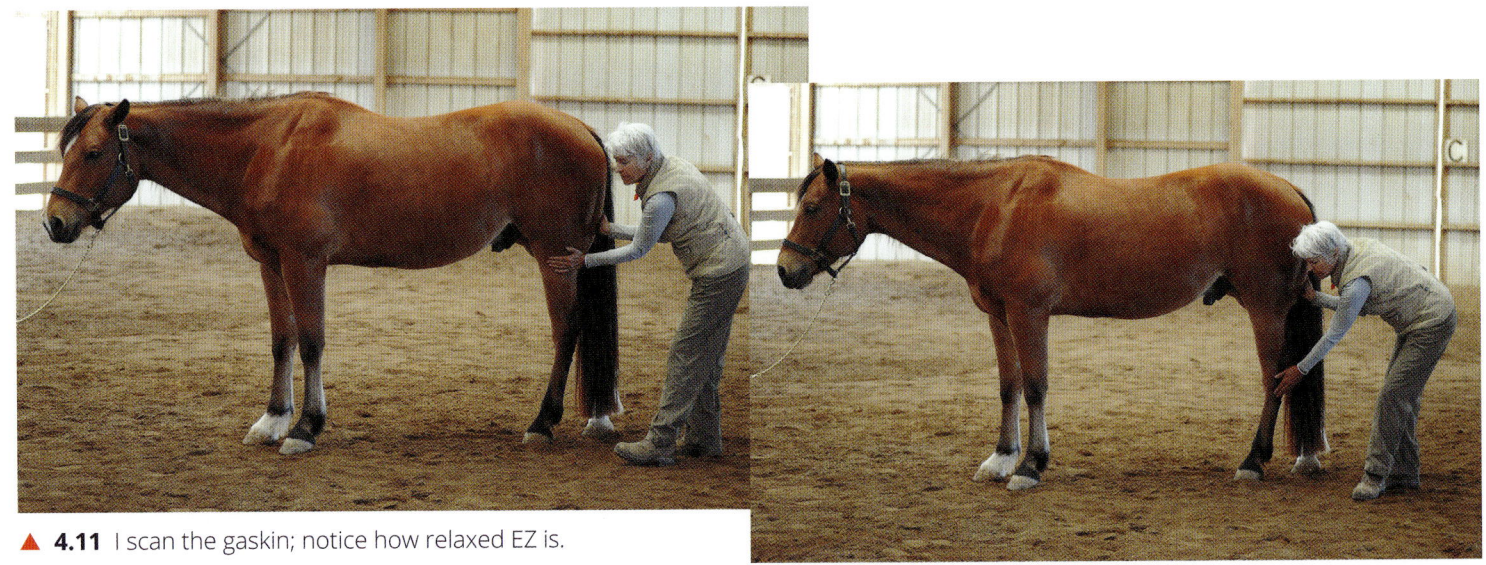

▲ **4.11** I scan the gaskin; notice how relaxed EZ is.

▲ **4.12** The hock can be a sensitive area; my contact is at the horse's approval. I can offer the contact later, again.

▶ **4.13** Most horses approve of tail contact when initiated without force. Sensitivity to tail contact is a clue to hind end imbalance.

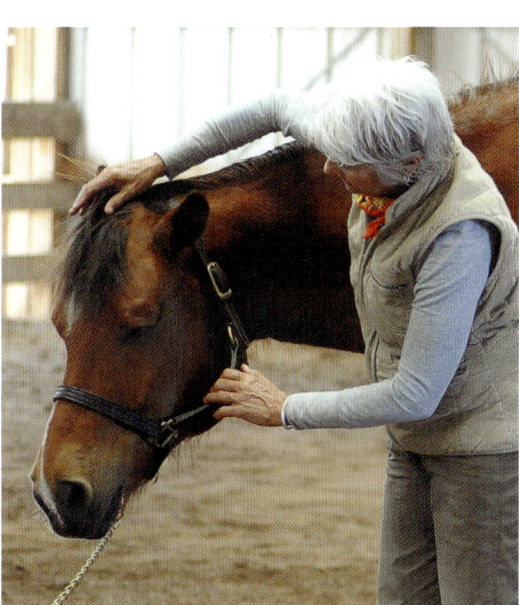

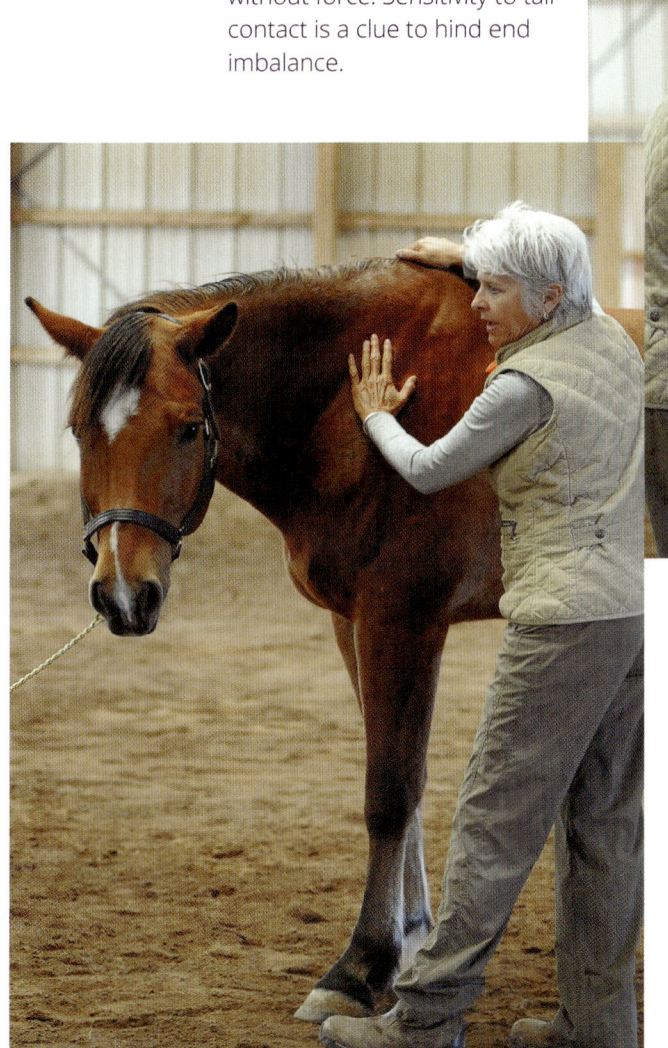

▲ **4.14** EZ drops into a Still Point in the body scan. The horse changes even during the scan! This soft, flowing scan can be part of handling routines and create easy, progressive changes for the horse.

◀ **4.15** This poll change on EZ looks like nothing is happening. We know that horses don't relax like this with deep attention unless it's worth their time! Again, I never interrupt a Still Point change.

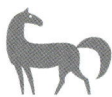

of how your touch feels. You adjust your hand speed for the horse's comfort. With practice, the scan helps find new problems and keeps track of old strains and injuries.

With this basic contact on the horse's body, you are checking in on his tolerance for contact that day, and looking for anything that might have changed for him. You use your palms for the scan.

How to Scan

Here is a list of the main things to remember when scanning the horse:

- With flat palms, sweep the horse's body, following the hair direction.
- Keep the fingers soft and flexible, adjust speed to suit the horse.
- Begin in an area that suits the horse best.
- Flow in the direction of the hair.
- Follow body contours, feeling as much sensation as possible.
- A fluid hand without stops allows the horse to drop into a deep awareness.
- Hands should be warm enough to feel the tissue.
- Notice the areas that interest the horse most.

> When the horse reacts with displeasure, stop and adjust the hand contact. Options include working in a different area, going much softer, or ending the session. Choose easy areas before working on sensitive, chronic, problem areas.

Information to Absorb When Scanning

- Does the skin have slide and some freedom and movement?
- Is the skin tight, dense, or stiff?
- Does the horse react with irritation to the contact? This is often a stiffness clue.
- Has the muscle group become rigid? Larger or smaller?
- Is the mane's hair short, sparse, or ragged? This is a clue to tight neck fascia.
- Is the tail short? This indicates a tight dock and tail fascia.
- Rough, uneven hair anywhere on the horse indicates circulation problems.

Where You Will Begin Fascia-Change Work

After the scan, you will be able to choose a place on the horse's body to begin the work. Due to the scan, you will now know which areas interest the horse most. Where his body sank down or where he paid close attention to your hands are good places to start because you know these are where the horse feels good about your contact.

Types of Hand Contact

Many kinds of hand contact successfully change fascia; it's practical to use what works best for the horse and is most comfortable. A particularly hard area, such as the shoulder, needs repeated palm contact, then, suddenly—*whoosh*—it melts and releases giving the horse much needed relief. Intuition is a reliable guide as you explore your horse and his changes. Unlike human patients, horses react quickly and forcefully when something hurts them. All your contact must account for their stiffness and level of tolerance.

Palms

A palm melts adhesions and rigid areas without pain (figs. 4.16). It's also sensitive enough to feel the surface tissue easily. Let your palm melt the tissue, so the fascia has time to change. It's the heat that changes fascia. A palm works well on any sensitive area, as well as the forehead, knees, fetlock, and dock.

A palm appears passive, like nothing is happening, but it brings more heat to the fascia than other contact types. For a stiff horse, a palm accomplishes miracles with rigid tissue. A palm is especially good for stifles, abdominals, and foreheads. Less is more.

A hard area responds very well to sustained palm heat, especially until the tissue has enough "give" to allow stretching to increase the range of movement. Often, it's very stiff at first and the horse enjoys your warm palm more than stretching stiff fascia.

The palm is the best approach to a stiff barrel, abdominals, flanks, stifles, and spine. Hips are also often very tight, especially the hip point. Cup the hip point in your palm and hold for minutes; this brings good results. This area responds well to repeated releases: it's a dense, large area and the layers of fascia rise to the surface as you repeat palm contact here.

Soft Fist

This works well on the hindquarters and barrel (figs. 4.17 & 4.18).

Knuckles

Knuckle strokes should be used cautiously since they can feel too hard. They are commonly used on the ribs (fig. 4.19).

Stroke Patterns

Slow strokes help the fascia move when it's supple enough to follow the hand. Upward strokes help to release the gravity pull. You can vary speed and how you use your hands in these strokes, as the horse permits. Most Conformation Balancing strokes move in the

Wind : A Unique Response

Wind didn't like slow careful scans. His history didn't include much handling or grooming. His body was lean and muscular, with little fat or padding. A 16-hand, five-year-old gelding, he could hardly stand still when we went slowly over his body. Rapid "sweeping" was his choice. His entire first session was unusually brisk. The scan also indicated that he couldn't tolerate a soft deep stroke. We used a firm touch and stayed in areas where he tolerated the contact best. This first session succeeded on Wind's terms. His rider found him easier to tack up after one session and continued to help him progress.

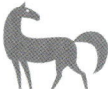

TYPES OF HAND CONTACT

▶ **4.16** Here, I melt the fascia with my palm. The fascia web network guarantees that this "site" will transmit change throughout the horse! A palm offers the horse maximum heat in dense, very stuck areas such as the back, sacral juncture and dock. The warmer the hands are, the better the results.

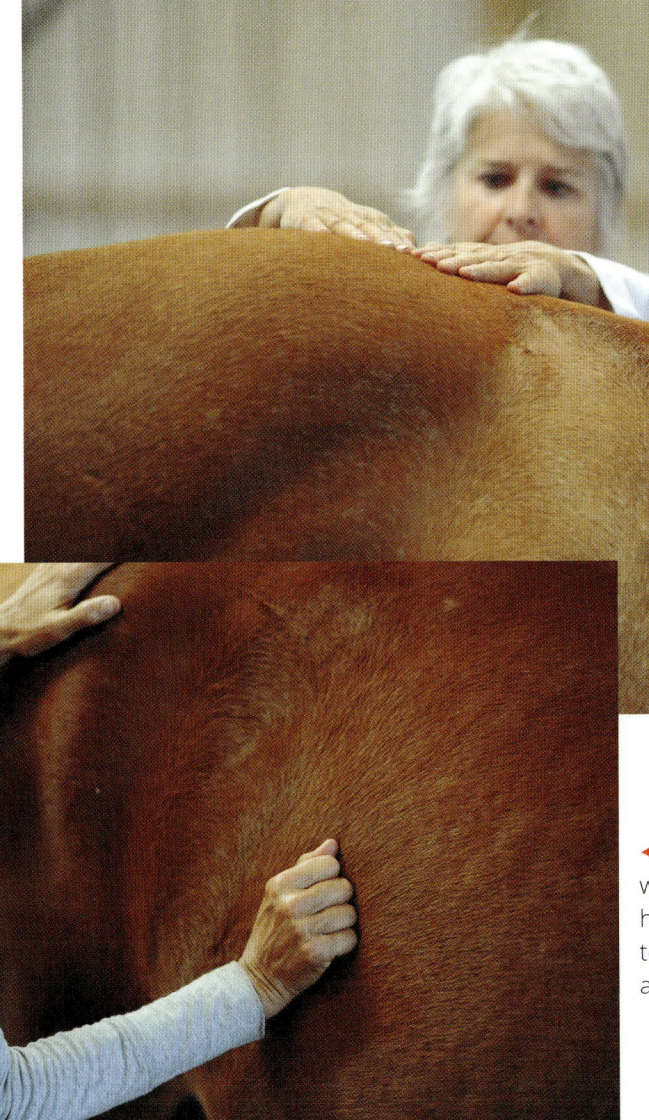

◀ **4.17** A soft fist works well in dense areas of the horse. If the horse objects to one kind of contact, I adjust quickly to another.

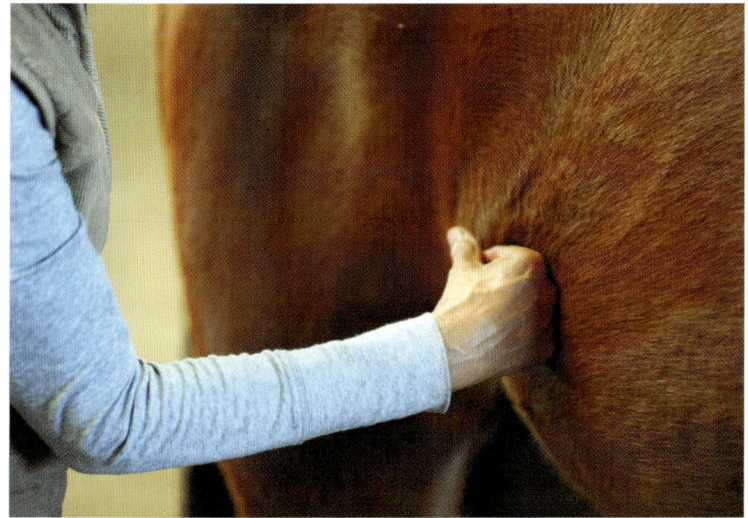

▲ **4.18** A soft fist lets me sweep the barrel, flanks, or stroke up the shoulders. Care in using my body properly saves human wear and tear.

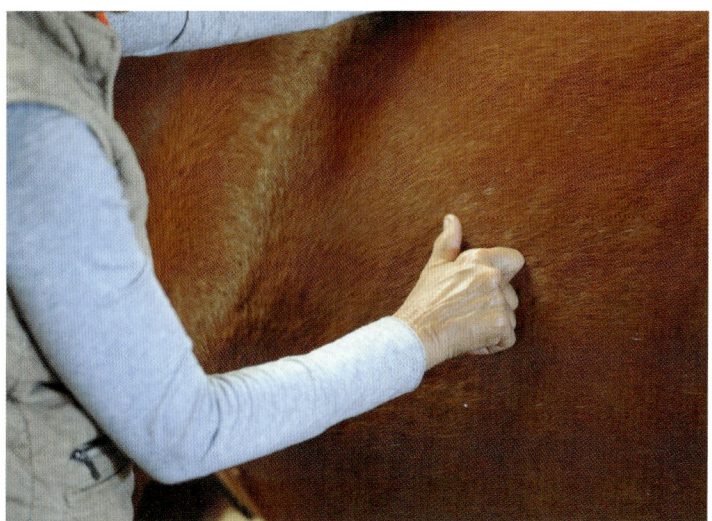

▲ **4.19** My knuckles work well in the intercostal muscles (ribs) if the horse is soft enough. When he's stiff, he'll object and my palms work better.

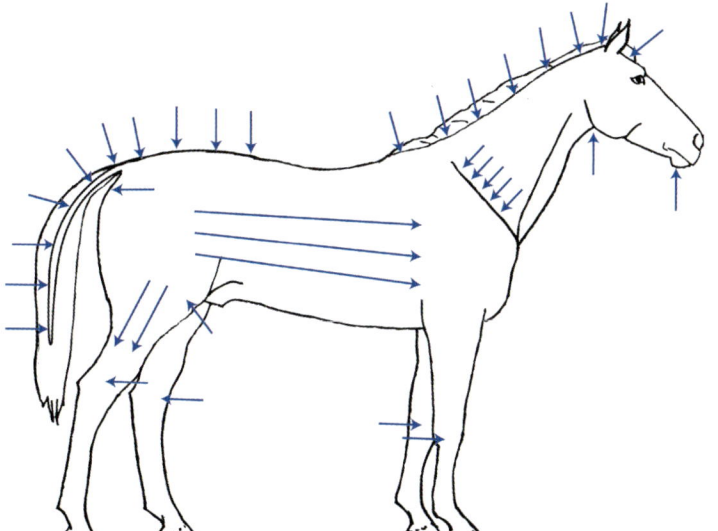

▲ **4.20 A** Stroke patterns: This art shows the different directions fascia can move to gain more range and flow. The direction varies. You can use whatever hand contact suits the horse in these direction patterns. Also, allow your own intuition to guide you.

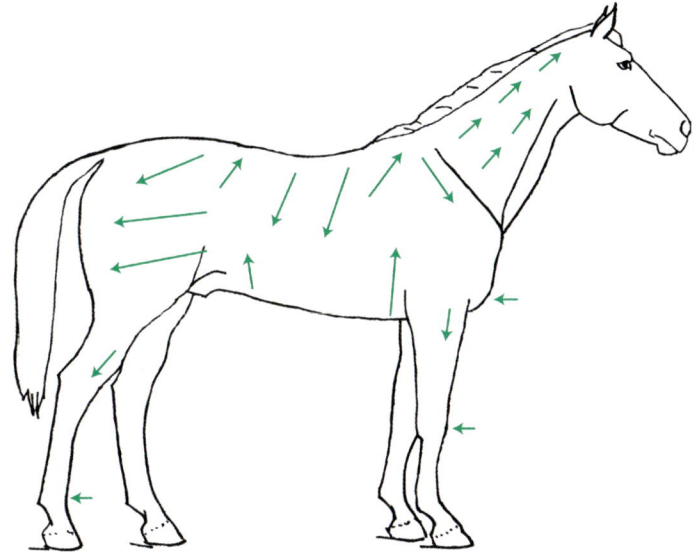

▲ **4.20 B** Stroke patterns: Upward strokes are effective since they help release the effects of downward gravity pull. It is helpful to stroke up, sometimes specifically in the areas depicted here.

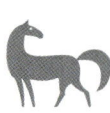

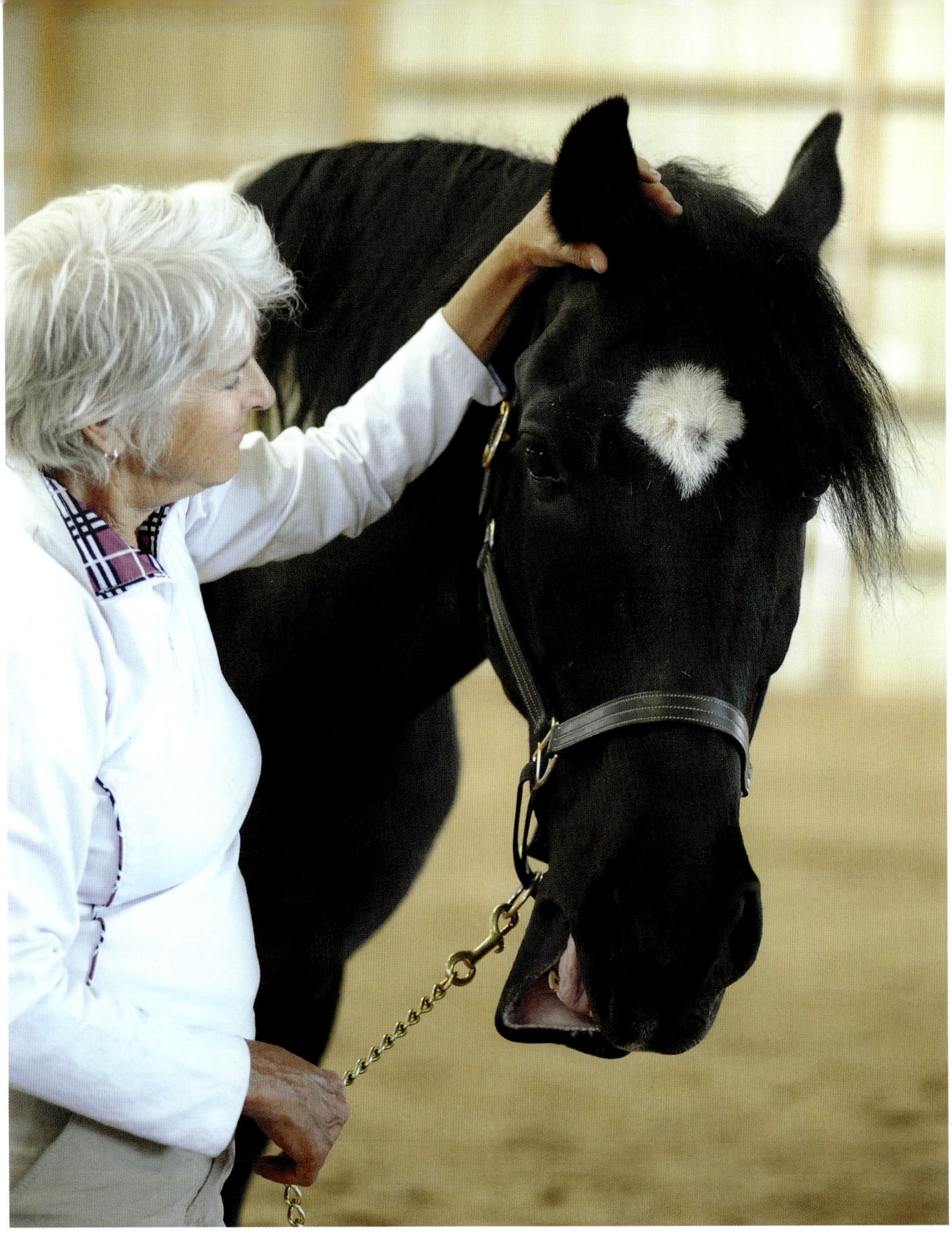

▶ **4.21** Beau licks and chews in his ear change. His right ear is tighter than the left. My thumb and finger sink gently into the fascia. This is an excellent change to offer the horse regularly.

direction of the horse's hair, as you do during the body scan. When stroking up the barrel, you go vertically on the horizontal hair growth (this does not irritate the horse). At the end of a balancing session, an organizing stroke from the horse's dock to his poll (against the hair) can be done with the palm. This is a slow stroke done in one long sweeping motion. It allows the fascia to flow better from the front to back of the horse. Often, the horse stretches out and lowers his neck as he enjoys this organizing stroke. The illustrations (figs. 4.20 A & B) are directional guides when the horse is supple enough. Stiff horses, particularly old horses, find strokes too painful at first; you can use the directional strokes with these horses after they have enough fascia balance. The key is to follow the horse's approval.

Stretching the Fascia

Here, move your hands gently in different directions to create a motion that feels pleasant to the horse. This gentle twisting motion of the palms is effective in dense areas like the sacral juncture and neck crest. It can also be used on the back, along the spine and withers. We use this twisting motion as the horse approves. If the horse is stiff, the fascia must melt first for this to be comfortable. The gentle twist helps release the fiber adhesions.

Exploring the Horse's Body

Once you've practiced the scan and different hand contact methods, it is time to explore basic areas on the horse. Start at the horse's head.

Head, Poll, and Neck

The body's remarkable ability for self-repair shows in head, poll, and neck changes for the horse. The horse is usually very receptive here because he feels so much better immediately. He may have suffered with headaches for years, perhaps since an accident at six months of age. A horse with an old injury to the head will happily stand quietly for many sessions that bring him relief. Occasionally, he'll need a break and "flick you away" to digest his change.

When the poll is unbalanced, the scan reveals an uneven or tipped-forward structure. The variation is infinite, but you'll feel the changes. It's common for the poll to shift extremely on its way to balance. Don't be concerned about it. You keep offering the contact until the horse isn't interested or he flicks you away.

The neck always requires change. Most necks are stiff and benefit from melting fascia on the line of the crest, as well as toward the poll area. Time spent here is well rewarded with a progressive neck flexion and lengthening. The neck also improves with the shoulder-crease openings, which I explain in chapter 5 (p. 91).

Ears

The ears are a "miracle area" for helping horses (figs. 4.21 & 4.22). Many have experienced trauma around the base of the ear as well as the entire ear, up to the tip. This can be caused by tight-fitting tack, or head strain. A gentle and effective technique is to hold the ear very softly. Once the horse understands you aren't squeezing or grabbing at his ear, he relaxes and enjoys the changes. As your thumb sinks into the base of the

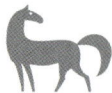

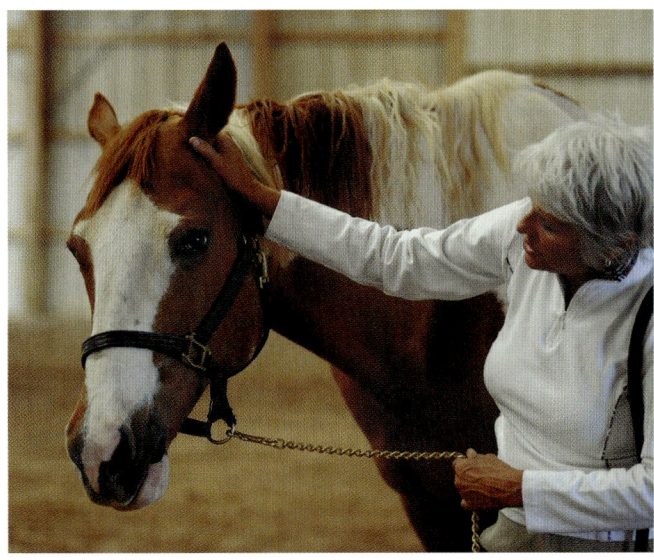

▲ **4.22** Scout happily sinks into his change in this ear release; Scout had strain resulting from his jumping career.

ear, head changes occur. These releases often last many minutes and bring great relief from anxiety. One ear usually needs much more attention than the other. When you offer these often, the emotional progress for the horse is rapid.

Jaw

The jaw is another important area. Look to see if the horse is uneven in his jaw from side to side. In many, one side of the jaw is larger. This adds to poll and head imbalance. It also hinders eating, despite good dental care.

Slip your fingers into the space under his jaw and sink the fingers upward (fig. 4.23). Put a palm on his cheek and wait for changes. Cup your hand behind his jawbone, sinking into the fascia of the jaw. Let the

space open and a whole new jaw may emerge along with a new, delicate, muzzle profile. Use the fingers to melt the space along his jawbone; as it opens wider, his throatlatch will deepen. This gives more space for neck flexion.

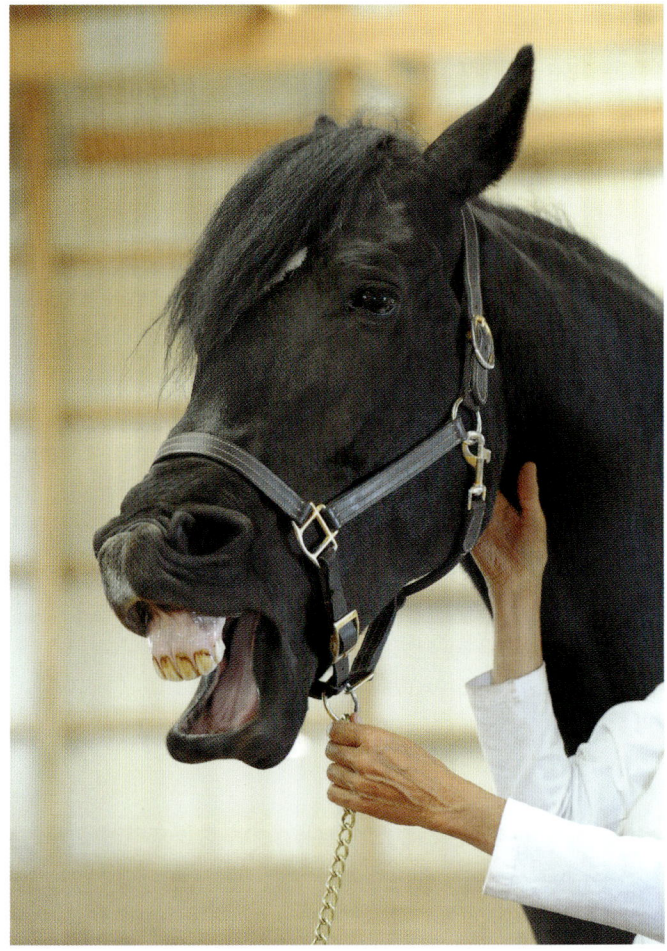

▲ **4.23** Beau is in Still Point here as my fingers sink up into his jaw fascia. A tight jaw creates a lot of mental tension for the horse, and being collected is painful for him. Although he's yawning, notice the "inner" look in his eye.

Follow the Sensations

Your palms and fingertips give you accurate tissue information if you trust what you feel is happening. Earlier, I mentioned that heat release tells me that the fascia strain is old and extensive. As your hands learn to differentiate the different levels of fascia strain, you learn to "chase the changes."

With a warm hand, the fascia spread is easy to feel (fig. 4.24). A sign of deep change is heat—it rises to your hand, perhaps growing very hot and coming in waves. You may at times feel a sensation of pins and needles in your own hands as the horse's stuck fascia tissue returns to circulation. This is common with deep, old imbalances. These sensations pass. The horse usually is deep in Still Point when he's experiencing these kinds of releases.

Heat tells you how old the event was and how much strain it created. The heat may feel scorching; if so, after working, your hands can be cooled with water. All heat held in the fascia must be released for a complete change. In a dense large area, like a hindquarter, it takes repeated sessions for full change. Often, you get good results by moving your hands slightly in all the directions, opening the area to free movement.

Shoulders, hind end, and withers are all areas that usually require repeated sessions for full recovery. Think about it, a horse can weigh 1,100 pounds or more. It takes enough heat to melt the stuck fascia for connecting normally again. Extraordinary results surface after releasing compressed fascia, even though the horse is "resting" and not working actively to build muscle.

I try for three full releases from the horse before moving to another area. However, as some of the stories show, a horse may need an entire hour of change

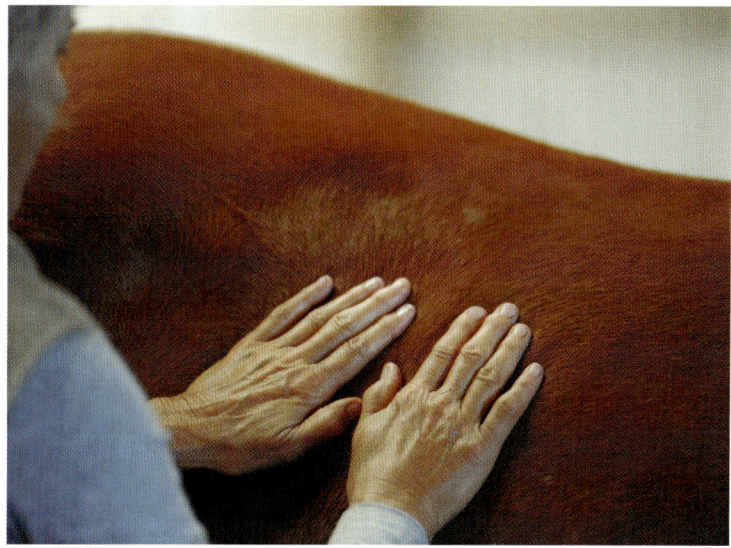

▲ **4.24** Your fingers become very sensitive. Here, EZ and I wait to feel the "melt" of fascia change. One sensation I get is a "worm-like" feeling of the fascia moving under the skin.

HEAD IMBALANCES

- Offset jaws in the muzzle profile; a jutting lower lip.

- Uneven eyes; one eye might even look larger or be set differently.

- Uneven nostrils, one may look farther back or higher.

- Uneven forehead bones.

- A "dent" or other "impact area" in the face.

- Uneven occipitals or poll, one side is higher or more forward.

- One side of the jaw is thicker than the other.

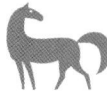

in one area in a first session. You follow the horse to guide you here. Sometimes, one kind of release often truly advances a horse past a miserable imbalance. The head changes are best offered many times, in whatever amount of time the horse agrees to. While it might seem endless, the balancing does come—and suddenly the horse won't be interested in further contact in that area. However, remember to return to it later in case there are more changes waiting.

Shoulders

The shoulder is the center of gravity; the shoulder muscles are not directly attached to the skeleton, and

this gives the horse's musculature an independent balance, like a four-wheel drive. Balanced conformation depends on a freely working shoulder. Observing the horse's shoulder structure can save you time hunting for solutions to hind lameness and other imbalances. Often, hind lameness results from shoulder imbalance, as some of the horse stories in this book show.

When you scan, the shoulder often feels hard and rigid, almost wooden. Tight or stuck shoulder creases and muscles will compress the neck and withers (fig. 4.25). Shoulder compression also creates tight elbow areas, which destroy the four-wheel-drive ability of a freely moving shoulder. When the shoulder creases are tightly closed and the elbows are also tight, the neck compensates by tightening and shortening as well. This makes the front of the horse rigid and unresponsive; he must drag the hind around. The barrel grows larger due to atrophy and the horse acquires a "light front and hind, and a large-paunchy-barrel look." This is an unbalanced horse for most riding, including hills, jumping, dressage, roping, and cutting.

Don't be discouraged by rigid, tight shoulders on the horse. They do respond to the change no matter how wooden they feel. You start with the shoulder knowing that the center of gravity must be functional for the horse to be balanced. The neck changes depend on the shoulder for space. This is an example of the interrelatedness of the body parts and how compensations affect conformation. When you look at bony high withers, it seems genetic, but it's often due to tight shoulders and cranial imbalance.

Withers are often mentioned because they are so important to the shoulder balance (fig. 4.26). Also, high withers are a common trait in many horses. In most

SENSATIONS FELT DOING FASCIA-CHANGE WORK

- Heat.

- A worm-like or rope sensation under the skin.

- A sheet of tissue rises under your hand like a wave.

- Pins and needles.

- Heat, then cooling.

- A wooden feeling in the tissue that "melts."

- A radiant-heat feeling that floods.

- Flowing sensations.

- A wiry tightness in a fascial thread (common behind the ears).

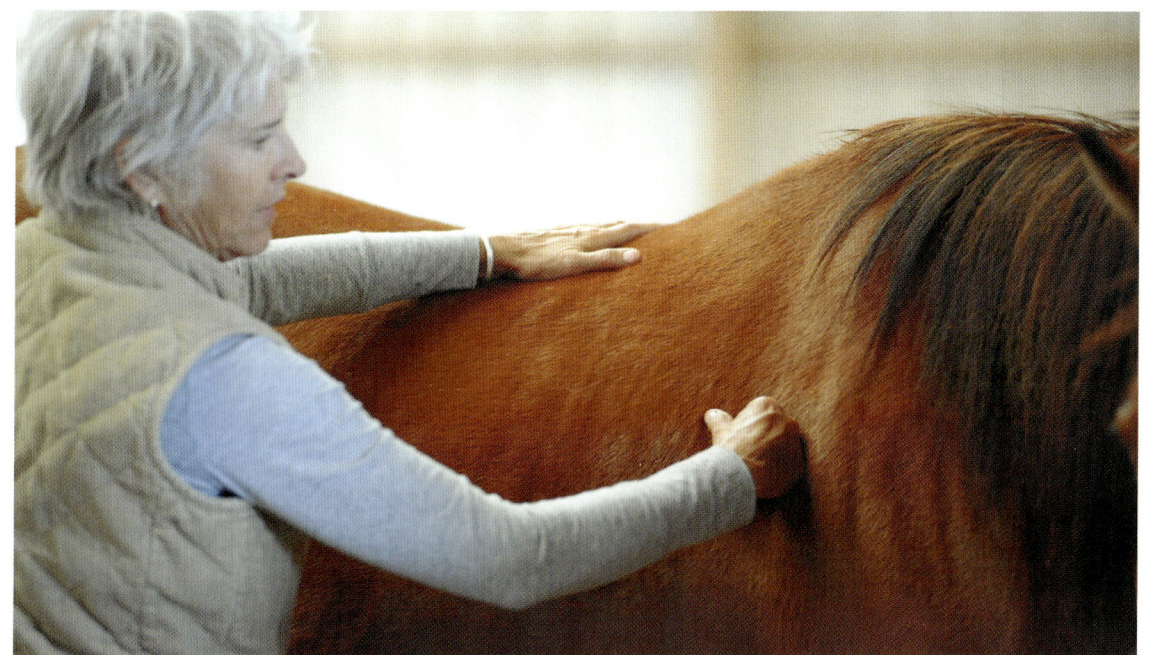

◄ **4.25** Shoulder creases require a sensitive approach. Here, a gentle prepping behind EZ's shoulder helps prepare him for accessing the crease. For many horses, the shoulder crease is an acquired taste. Once they understand the benefits, it is easy for them.

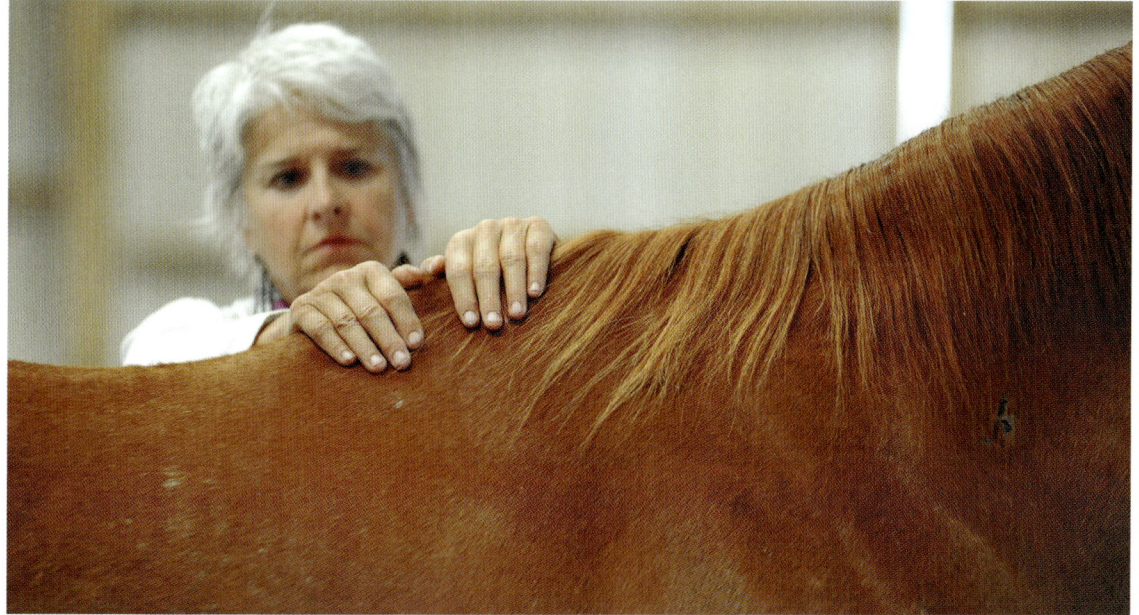

◄ **4.26** CT is our model here for the withers change release. The very stiff withers fascia open for wonderful changes to the shoulders and withers. These changes let the withers "spread," which may change saddle fit. While this looks very passive, the fascia is changing.

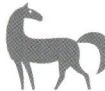

cases, however, these high, bony-looking withers aren't supported by well developed, supple shoulders. In this Conformation Balance work, the key areas that control conformation are emphasized. As the fascia-change work deepens, the neighboring areas also balance. As always, proceed at the horse's comfort pace and don't push for change he cannot yet accept. For a very stiff horse, opening the shoulder crease can require a few weeks of careful, patient contact.

With rigid, stuck shoulders, the horse can't maintain stability consistently: correct leads are inconsistent, if not impossible. Canters are lost. Stumbling is common. Lateral flexion and yielding are extremely difficult. Knee strain develops, too. In addition, horses with unbalanced, stuck shoulders are usually full of anxiety, despite a calm temperament. Shoulder imbalances make a horse fearful, which eventually create disturbances that force the rider to search for solutions. We go along, until we can't.

This work is all about following the stuck tissue and blockages to free the fascia for free movement. If you do all the releases needed, the problem resolves. Even with difficult shoulder imbalance, the horse can progress to being unrecognizable in less than a year.

Many riders assume that all the "hard" areas, particularly in the shoulder area, are muscle. They think this is a good thing for the horse, that is, he's "in condition." Actually, these hard places are often old strain areas with many adhesions. They are not productive, fit muscles anymore; they debilitate the horse since it becomes impossible for him to access them as active moving parts.

> The horse's shoulder is his center of gravity. Regular palm contact releases tight shoulder fascia, releasing the neck to build a crest.

As you touch the horse with a new awareness of fascia, you'll find these hard, stuck areas. When you look carefully, you'll often notice that the hard stiff shoulder that you thought was well-muscled, connects to a bony withers or flat neck. Then, you might remember that changing leads is very difficult. Suddenly, the hard shoulder is a different situation. This is how you connect the dots. The condition and connectivity of fascia affects the horse's performance.

Pectorals

A gentle hand is best when you contact pectorals. When they are different sized, this is a clue to strain. Your palm can make deep changes with soft, horizontal strokes. Also, you can sink your fingers gently to touch the sternum bone and wait for release there.

Barrel

Like a suspension bridge, the two ends of the horse are the structural anchors. The barrel keeps the two ends of the horse together. For this reason, it can become very strained and tight. A sore back is often traced to front and hind end imbalance. The barrel is the rib cage so as your flowing hands pass over it horizontally, you can feel how tight the ribs are (see the stroke patterns for the barrel on p. 61). Barrel strain is often the source of girthyness. Horses that are hard to saddle-fit often have fascial imbalance throughout their back and barrel.

Backs without muscle to protect and support the

spine are examples of how extreme strain has pulled the back tight. Paunchy, hanging barrels without enough abdominal support are another clue to imbalance. With barrel contact, notice if the coat is tight or if it is supple. This is a clue to fascial tightness: your fingers should be able to feel between the ribs easily, without digging. NOTE: Take care to be gentle in the posterior abdominal area—the place where predators would attack.

Elbows

I usually do elbow changes when I'm working on the barrel. Be aware that they are often very tight and the horse is very sensitive in the elbows. An open elbow is vital to shoulder stability. Usually, the elbow is stuck tight against the horse's ribs and chest. A good clue to elbow problems is the horse is girthy when being tacked up.

Slip your fingers into a tight elbow area to melt the space open (figs. 4.27 & 28). This change must be gentle and gradual. It helps to lean into the horse while using your inside hand to slide up between the elbow and rib area.

Often, there are strings of fascia and cords from strain as you sink upward into the "armpit" of the horse. Quick hard stops, jumping, front-end collection

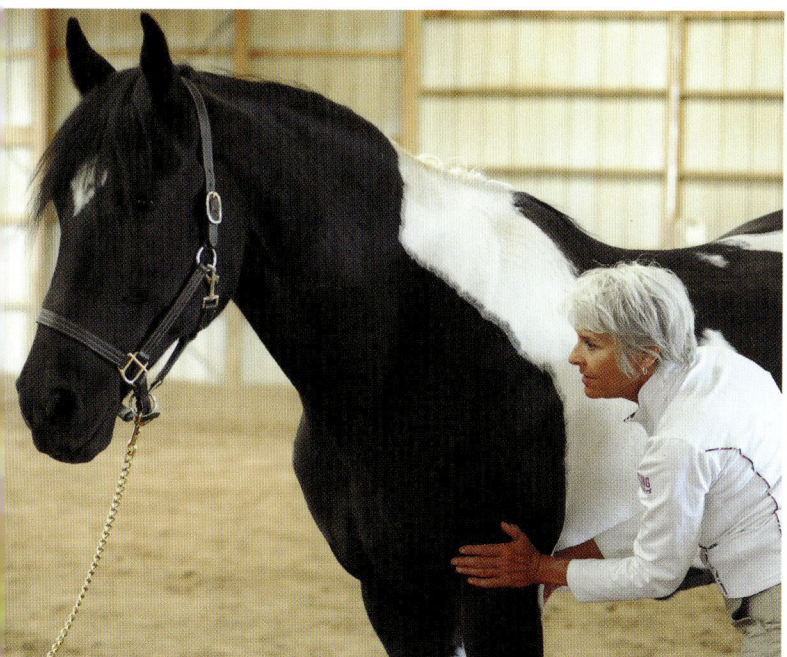

▲ **4.27** Elbows can't be overestimated for their role in shoulder freedom. I sink a soft hand up into Beau's elbow, waiting for it to open and offer space to the leg and shoulder.

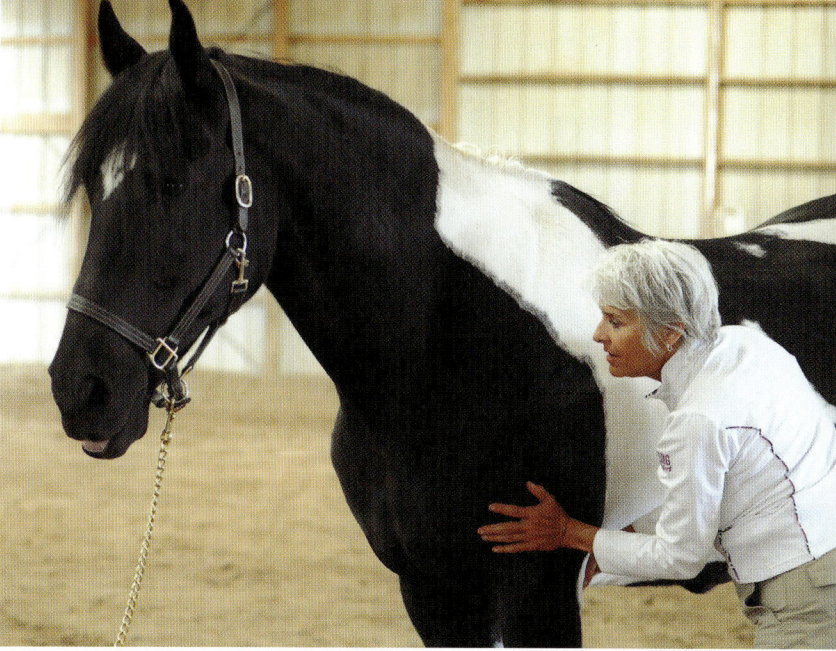

▲ **4.28** Beau shows a licking release as I sink up into his elbow space. When the elbow is tight, the shoulder will not fully open.

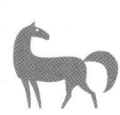

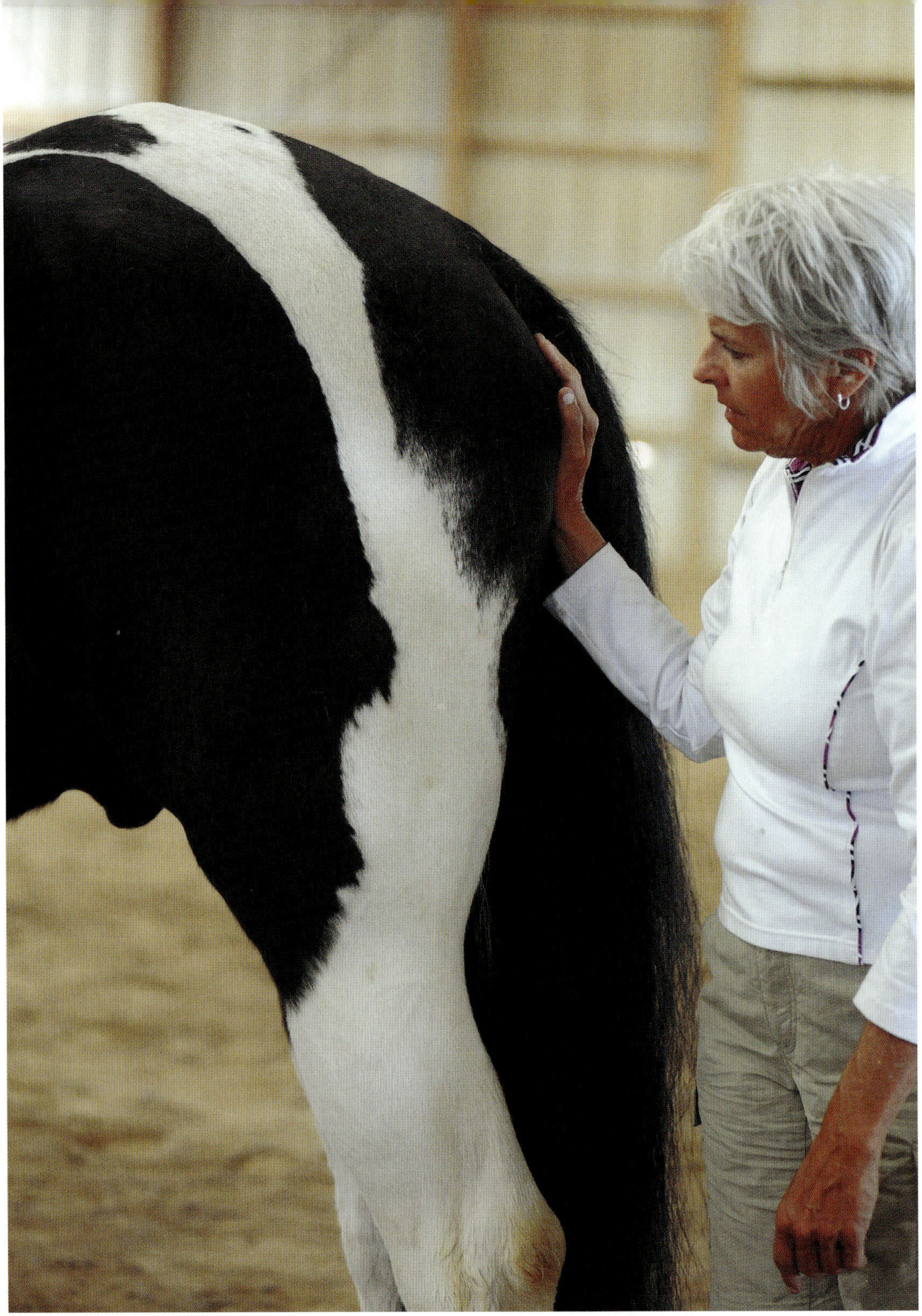

▶ **4.29** Beau models an ilium point change here. Apply this release to both sides. One side is always stiffer. Often, the stiffer ilium corresponds with a diagonal compensation in the head. For example, right ilium, left jaw, ear, or mouth compensation pattern.

techniques, and barrel racing tighten the elbow area more than average riding. You need to open this area repeatedly, for weeks at a time, to get complete change here. At times, it may take a few months. The gains include allowing complete freedom of the shoulder, which, in turn, raises the withers. When the elbow is wide open and easy to access, this indicates a free-moving shoulder.

The horse is often sensitive to elbow work at first, but he loves the relief. As the elbow opens, wider and deeper, contact is easier. Strides lengthen. Changing leads become easy. These changes are lasting and progressive.

Hindquarters

The large dense area of the hips and rump seems huge and it takes practice to develop sensitivity for feeling this large mass of body tissue. Don't be intimidated by its sheer size and mass. When you investigate here, you're looking for bony hips, lean flanks, and hollows anywhere. These underdeveloped areas tell you that fascia holding these large muscles and groups of muscles is compressed, which prevents the muscles from developing as needed for the horse's work. Due to the heat, a palm works well, despite its passive appearance.

The croup is usually tight and the dock is also an area that is compressed on most horses. In the hindquarters area, there are the hamstring, gaskin, and hock. Here, you're looking for "dents," injuries, or uneven proportions. Dents on the hind end are usually from being kicked. These dents deserve special attention with releases later in your work. Dents cause deep fascial disturbances that are actually not too difficult to resolve with some patient attention (figs. 4.29–4.31).

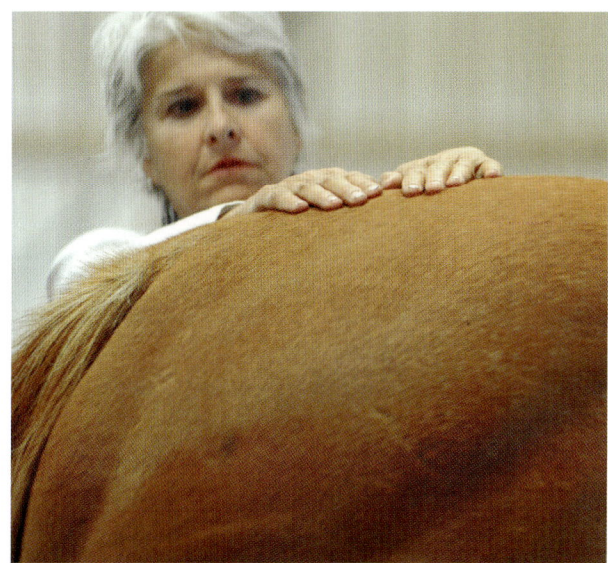

◀ **4.30** The croup is usually stiff. It's also a dense area that benefits from regular "melting" of the fascia, especially if you collect your horse.

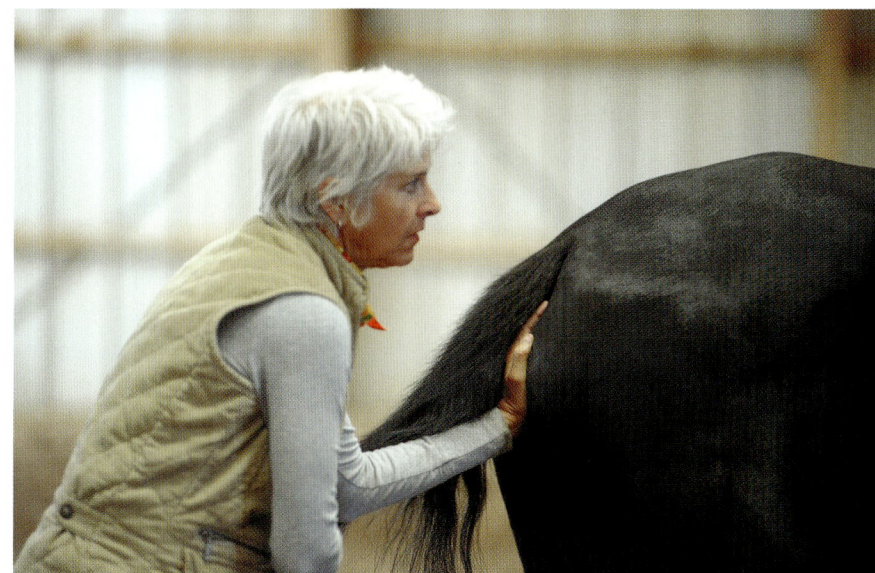

▲ **4.31** The ilium point, like our own "sitting-bones" point, is an area that brings much head to tail change benefit. Here, Jet lets me sink in at her ilium point.

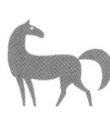

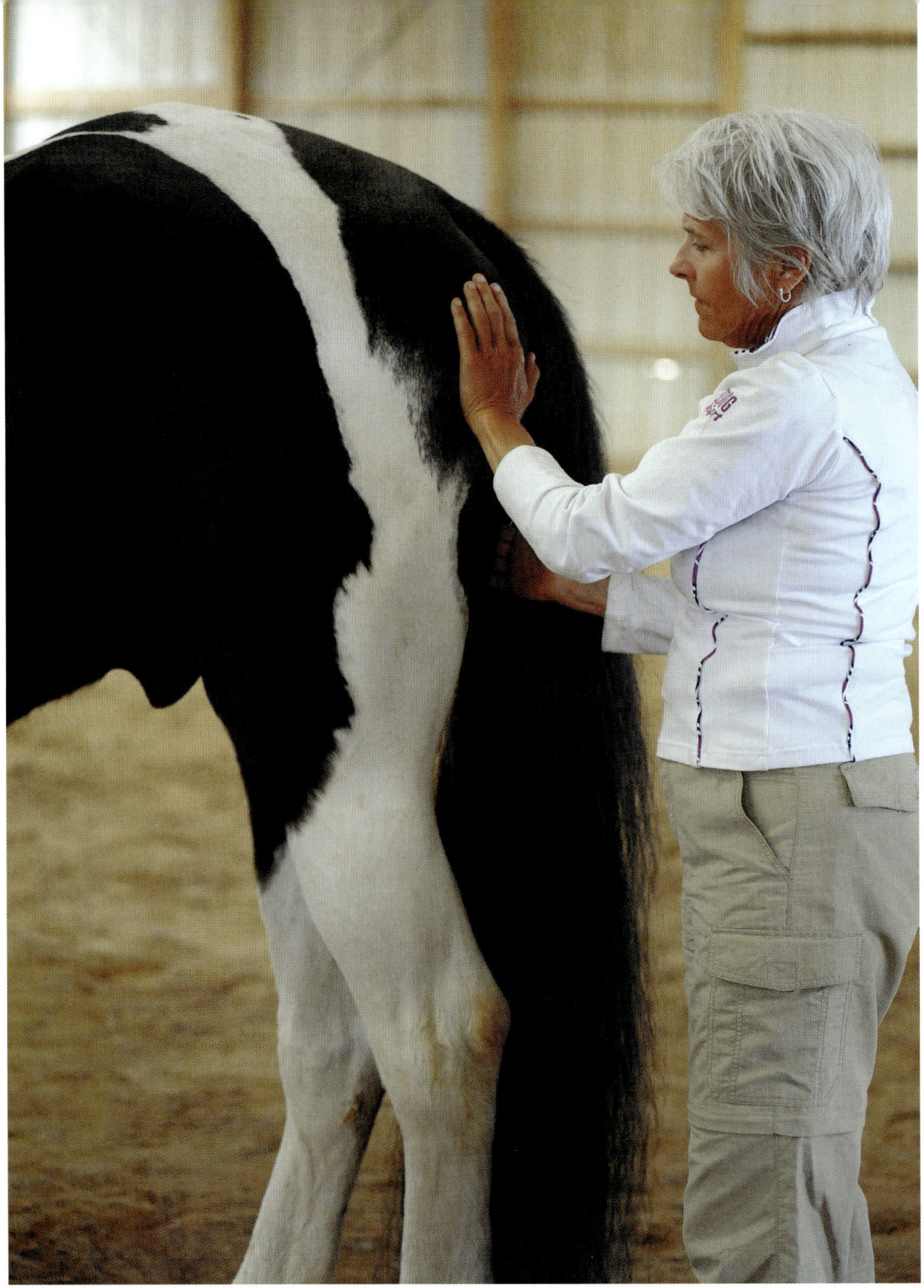

4.32 My right hand is sliding on Beau's adductor muscle. The source of pelvic imbalance leading to lameness is sometimes the pelvic floor, which is at the top, between the horse's legs.

Adductors

The adductors are the muscles on the inside of the horse's rear legs. Adductor strain often results from slipping in mud, snow, or ice. As you slide your hands slowly up to the top, where the horse's pelvic floor is, you may find a mass of mushy tissue or some hard stringy tissue. The mushy tissue is fascia piled up, and your hand contact melts it and allows it to spread. In time, mushy tissue clumps sometimes reveal hard, stiff adhesions. The stringy tissue is also from strain but more advanced in its adhesion-hardening progress, and more heat contact is needed to fully change it.

Smooth, fluid fascia is healthy fascia. Adductors are important for collection, jumping, and stopping. The horse usually stands with his rear legs tightly together when you begin work here; when he begins to feel better, he opens wide and it's easier to finish the changes (figs. 4.32 & 33).

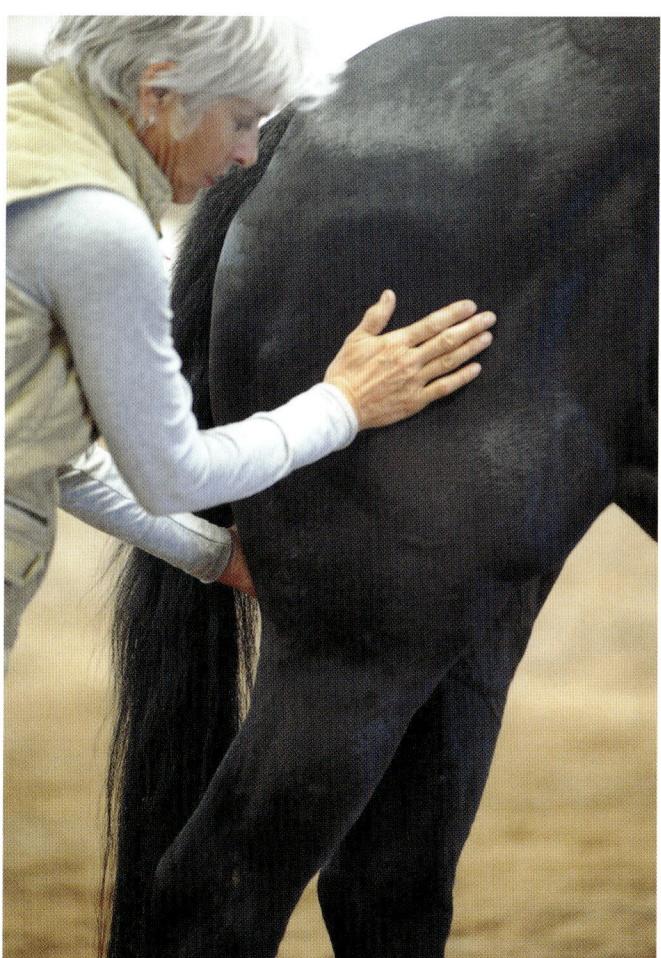

▲ **4.33** Jet stands quietly while I slide my left hand up the inside of her leg toward the adductors and pelvis.

Rocky: The Ultimate Stoic—Almost!

Rocky, a chestnut Quarter Horse, was a true stoic. He didn't respond with licking or chewing. None of the usual "approval cues" showed in the session. I knew fascia changes were happening, but he was not demonstrating release cues. I was working with his adductors when his owner called out: "Guess what? Rocky's drooling!"

So, the stoic had a productive first session, after all! Over a year, in monthly sessions, Rocky found more feeling in his hind end and shoulders. He became more flexible and less shut-down emotionally.

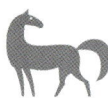

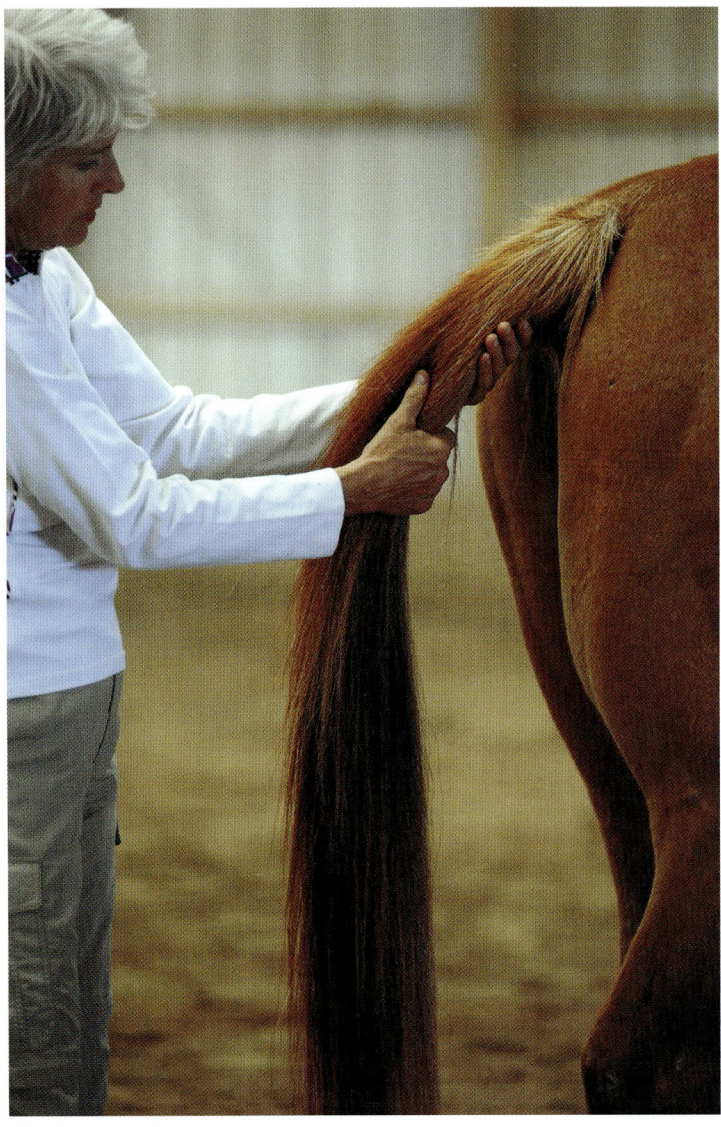

▲ **4.34** I hold CT's tail with my hands on the meaty part to melt the fascia. Horses like this and the results reward the effort! The tail often transforms the hindquarters.

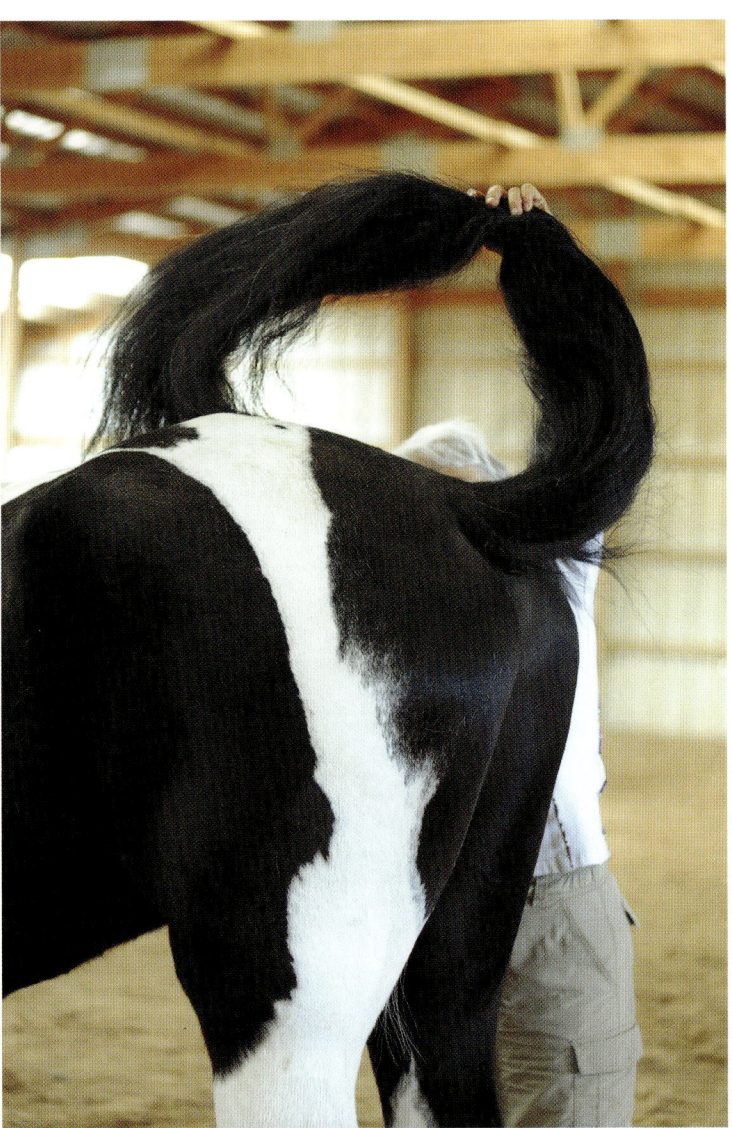

▲ **4.35** Beau models the tail lift here, letting me almost circle it. Beau's tail is unusually flexible.

Tail

The tail is a major part of the hindquarters puzzle. When you first handle it, the tail seems to have little muscle, yet it is essential to the horse's hindquarters freedom of movement. Tail releases for stiff tail vertebrae are wonderful paths to hindquarters progress. It's a miraculous change for such a huge dense area of muscle through a small, easy-to-handle part of the horse. An expressive tail is easy to notice.

The tail is the horse's coccyx. As you know, it's a painful injury when you fall on your tailbone. The horse uses his tail to balance. The tail is kept fluid by movement. Wild horses move a distance of at least 50 miles a day over varied terrain. A much more "sedentary" lifestyle means the horse's tail becomes less flexible: it loses articulation of the vertebrae.

Many tails are like broomsticks: they are stiff, unable to bend laterally, or curve upward. Very few tails are able to curl back to touch the croup, as they would if flexible. In most cases, the horse's tail can bend laterally somewhat and, perhaps, curl halfway up toward his croup, but that is all he can allow. Many horses are concerned when you begin to handle their tail at all.

Complete release of the tail is vital to maintaining head changes, which create so much improvement in self-carriage and collection (figs. 4.34–4.36). You can't spend too much time releasing a tail. Short opportunities bring good results, even when the horse snacks, or when we spend time companionably. The horse loves this change.

Tail Lifts and Holding the Tail

Here, you slowly lift the tail, curving it toward the croup (fig. 4.37). You stand to the side of the horse and not behind him. The range of lift increases with practice.

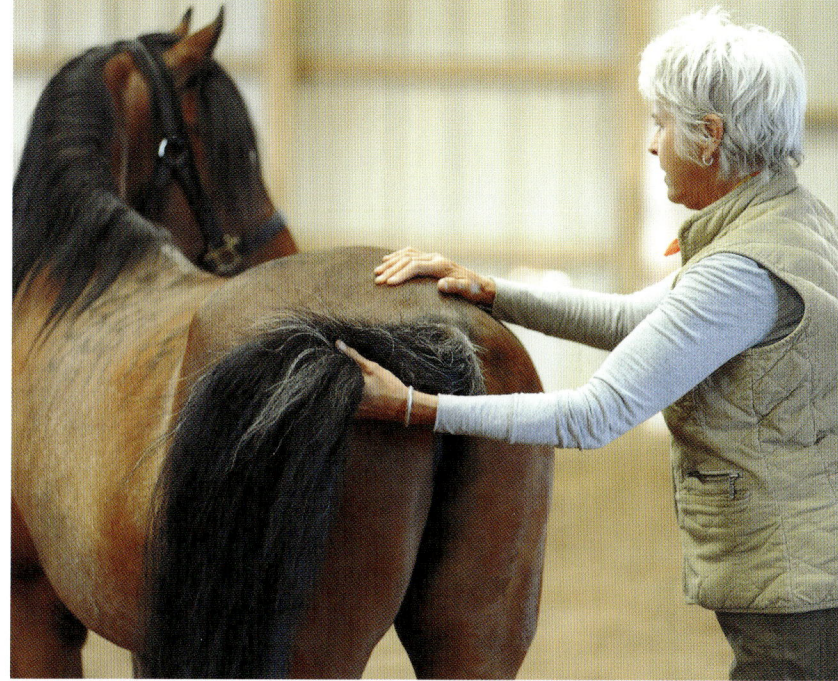

▲ **4.36** Samson, a Paso Fino, models a tail circle here. Tail dock changes are another hugely rewarding release, bringing progressive hind end flexion.

BENEFITS OF TAIL RELEASES INCLUDE:

- A plumed, relaxed tail.
- A free dock.
- Sacral freedom; lumbar freedom.
- Increased pelvic power and flexion.
- Better canter leads.

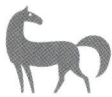

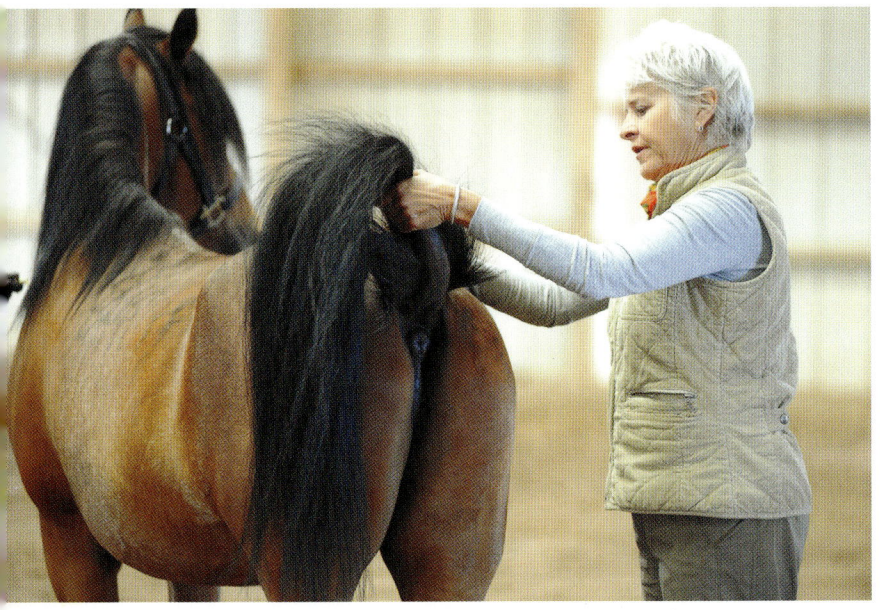

Three lifts are helpful. Hold it up as long as the horse's eye agrees he likes it. Sometimes this can last for a minute. After lifting, hold the tail between your hands, letting your skin contact the horse's skin as much as possible. Heat goes through the tail hair.

In minutes, this astonishingly simple key to hindquarters freedom brings an additional gain as the horse is again able to plume his tail in freedom. As you hold the tail, the head and poll are also balancing, since all areas are connected by the internet of fascia. Many surprising hindquarters changes are accelerated by tail changes, including change in the entire sacral/lumbar area. Tail work is a very beneficial, regular routine for hindquarters maintenance.

Tail Rotations

Gently rotate the tail three times in each direction. This is a good pre-ride exercise. As the horse permits, gently raise it to a vertical. Notice whether the vertebrae can articulate or if they are rigid, and whether sections of the tail lack flexibility. The more time spent to gently release the tail, the more freedom you create for the entire sacral area.

Tail Pull

You can include the tail pull immediately, if the horse likes it. The tail pull is another excellent pre-ride stretch. Here, you stand behind the horse, making sure you can see one of his eyes, and hold the tail in your hands, but not wrapped around your hand. Slowly lean back until your full weight is pulling against the horse. The horse often angles himself for the best stretch (fig. 4.38).

Leo: Respect Required

When working on an accomplished Welsh pony at a horse show, I decided to change hands for a better position on his neck. As I lifted my hand from Leo in mid-stroke, he turned and glared at me, "How dare you interrupt my relief?" his eyes said. The owner and her young daughter looked at me, and exclaimed. "Look at his face!" I admitted that my interrupting his neck change was a huge irritation to him and apologized to all.

In this single session for a fit horse that was performing well and winning ribbons, we can still see how our hand contact must respect the horse and what he is feeling.

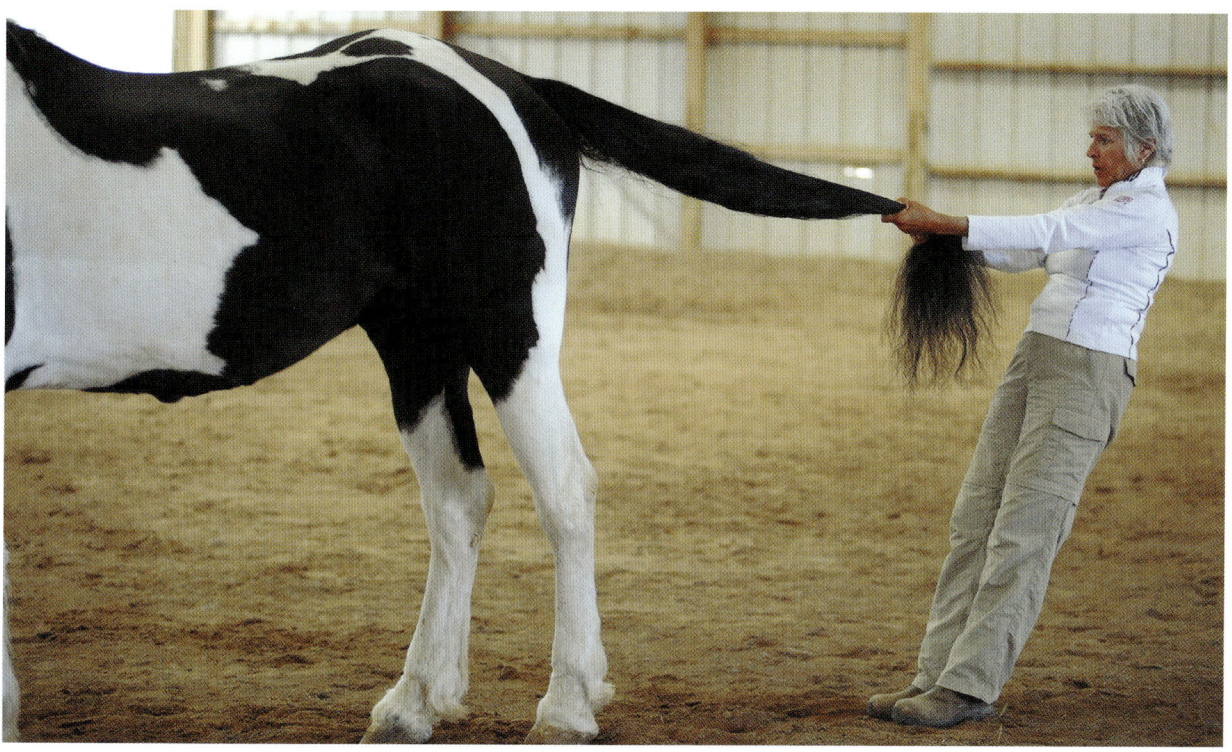

◀ **4.38** Beau leans away from me in his tail pull. I watch his eyes and ears for safety. I do not wrap his tail around my hand. This stretch improves the topline and is a tonic for the horse.

TIPS FOR A BODY SCAN AND BALANCING SESSION

- Vary each session length according to whatever the horse permits. Short sessions of 15 minutes are very effective for young horses. Longer sessions of an hour or more suit the stiff and older horse. The more problems the horse has, the more he likes longer sessions. As he improves, he doesn't need continual intensive contact.

- Use contact with both the front and hind ends of the horse.

- Address as many parts of the horse as possible to prevent a residual "jam."

- Life is full of exceptions. If a horse enjoys a poll release—and chooses nothing else—this is perfect.

- A tail-to-head organizing stroke unites the horse after many changes. Here, you sweep your palm from the dock along the horse's topline, going slowly and against the hair, all the way to the poll.

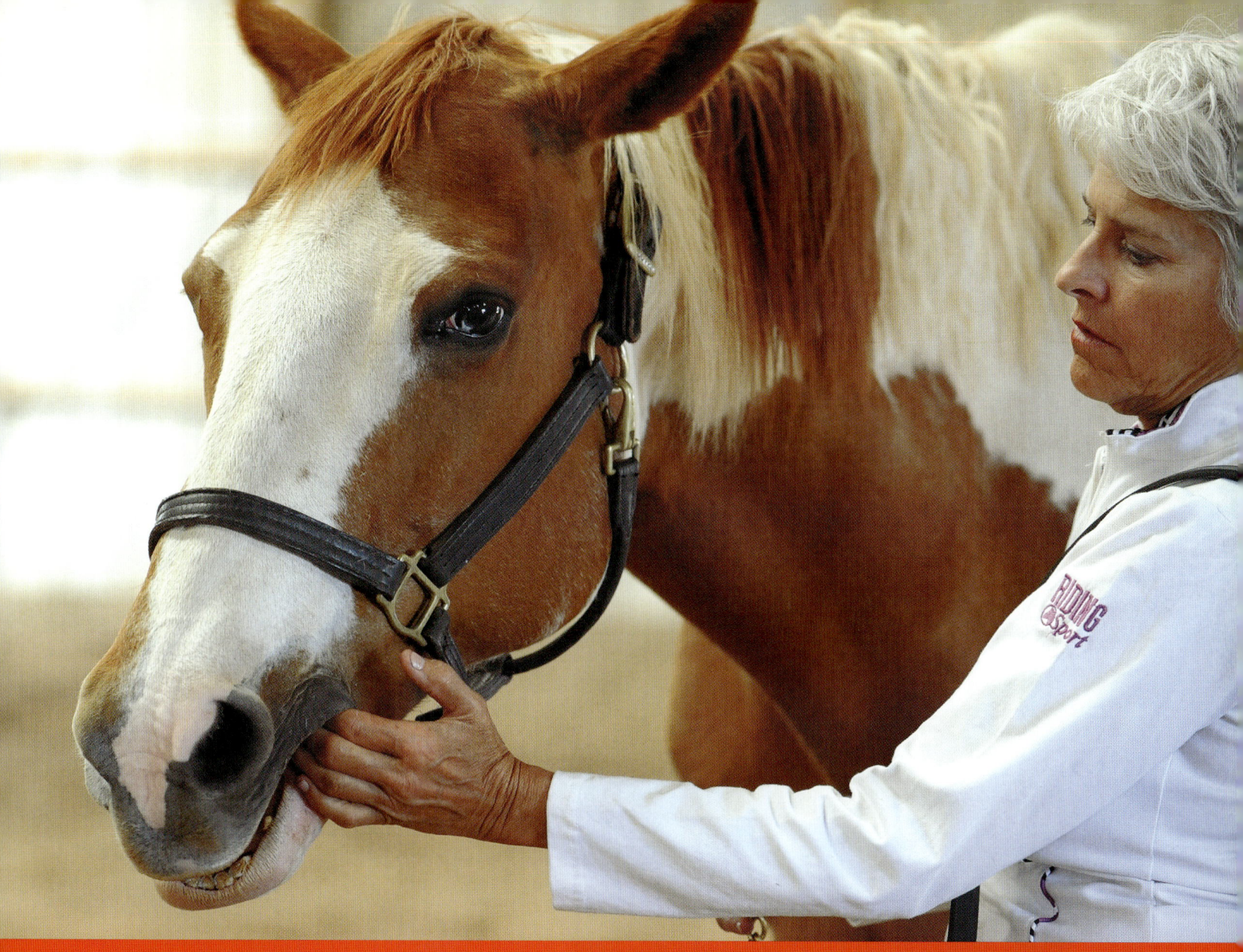

5 | Deeper Transformations

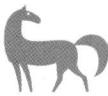

The Horse's Head

In Conformation Balancing, you are often working with the horse's head. Throughout this book, you will see many pictures of head balancing, and these examples show how intently the horse focuses during head changes. Tack directs and controls his head movements, and this alone should remind us why we need to understand how well his head is balanced—or not.

Head balancing brings a great relief of anxiety. Imagine the wear and tear on the horse's head and neck from the moment of being started in the halter. Single-line longeing, a widely used practice when starting the young horse, is extremely stressful on the horse's

balance. The real problem is the tension placed on his poll and jaw, as well as the neck. This common training method may compromise the horse for the rest of his life with anxiety and inability to focus.

Poll structure is unique for each horse. Some polls are flat and feel like a solid single bone. Others have two peaks. Still other polls have one large peak in the center. As you learn to feel your horse—and other horses—you'll see how the poll moves and changes. Variations for horses are infinite: you may feel the poll move forward, backward, then up or down. This is all good. The hand is always soft and there is no pushing down on the horse. When the horse flicks you off, he's not interested—you can ask again later (figs. 5.1–5.4).

Common Causes of Head Imbalance

There are many common causes of head imbalance, including:

- Trailer injury and ceiling impact.
- Tying accident with a pullback incident.
- Single-line longeing.
- A birth accident (landing on the head, for example).
- Kick in the head from rough social behavior.
- Head injury from fencing or other grazing accident.

The forehead, or frontal bones, can be misaligned by a kick, head impact, birth event, or accident. The horse's eyes appear strained. The forehead may be uneven or there may be a mound or a dent. Your palm on the forehead balances it. This area may feel quiet, but it brings impressive change to the horse, and it often requires

FASCIA CHANGES ARE THE SHORTCUT

It's important to mention that distracting the horse with food, scented oils, or commotion prevents changes. There really are no shortcuts with fascia changes—it either changes or it doesn't. While fascia is self-intelligent, it is necessary for the horse to identify and complete the change. It is also necessary to allow the horse to finish all the changes needed by waiting for the lick-and-chew signal that the change has ended—without treats. If the horse doesn't identify the new relief, you are not finished yet.

HEAD BALANCING

▶ **5.1** Beau cocks one ear forward and one back as he intently receives this poll change. Notice how soft my hand looks as if it's just draped over his poll. Less is more; no pressure or pushing works here.

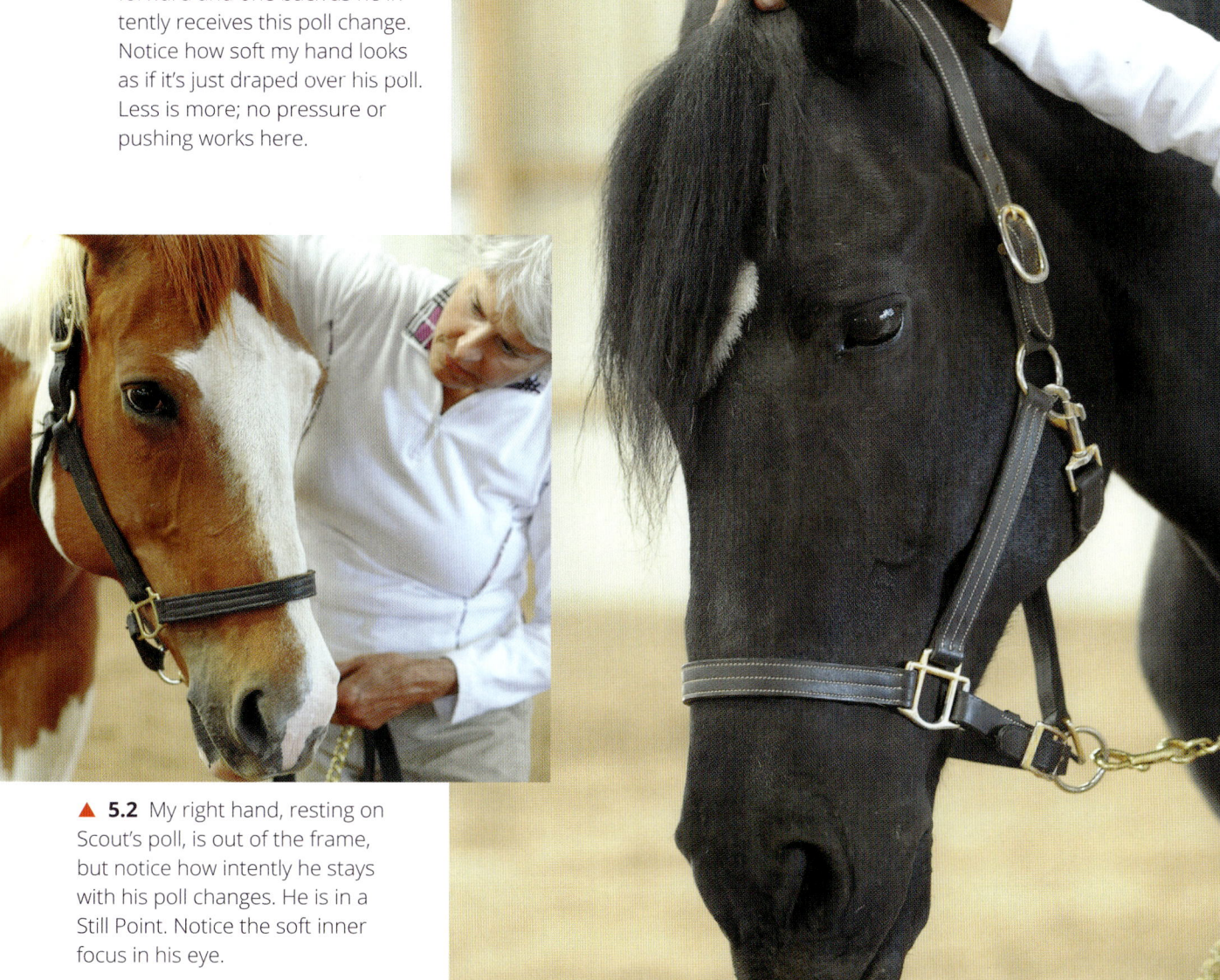

▲ **5.2** My right hand, resting on Scout's poll, is out of the frame, but notice how intently he stays with his poll changes. He is in a Still Point. Notice the soft inner focus in his eye.

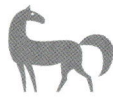

HEAD BALANCING (CONTINUED)

▶ **5.3** Beau drops his head for a poll change. The horse often drops lower, sometimes to a foot off the ground in this balancing change. My hand is draped almost casually on his poll.

▼ **5.4** Remy enjoys a Still Point as his poll balances.

more than a few sessions. Short sessions are perfect for these fascia changes (figs. 5.5 & 5.6).

A Magical Change for the Horse

As you practice feeling the horse's poll and sinking your fingers gently into the areas around his ears, the horse goes into an internally focused awareness. He is paying complete attention to his inner changes and his eye is inward. As the horse becomes conscious of his changes, and accepts feeling those changes, the changes deepen.

Like the tail, the head changes offer prompt progress to the horse's appearance. Dramatic changes in head shape, eye shape, and muzzle are common with head changes. Still Points last long minutes and come frequently (figs. 5.7–5.10). Head changes are

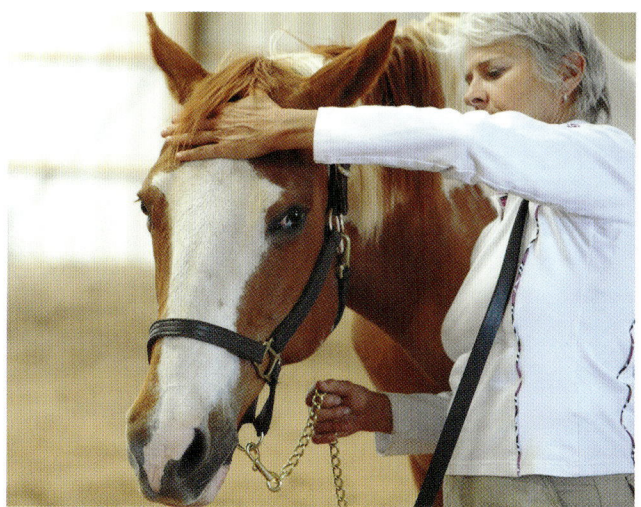

▲ **5.6** Scout is deep in Still Point in this forehead release. This area seems almost too obvious, yet many horses bang their foreheads into fences and during trailer loading.

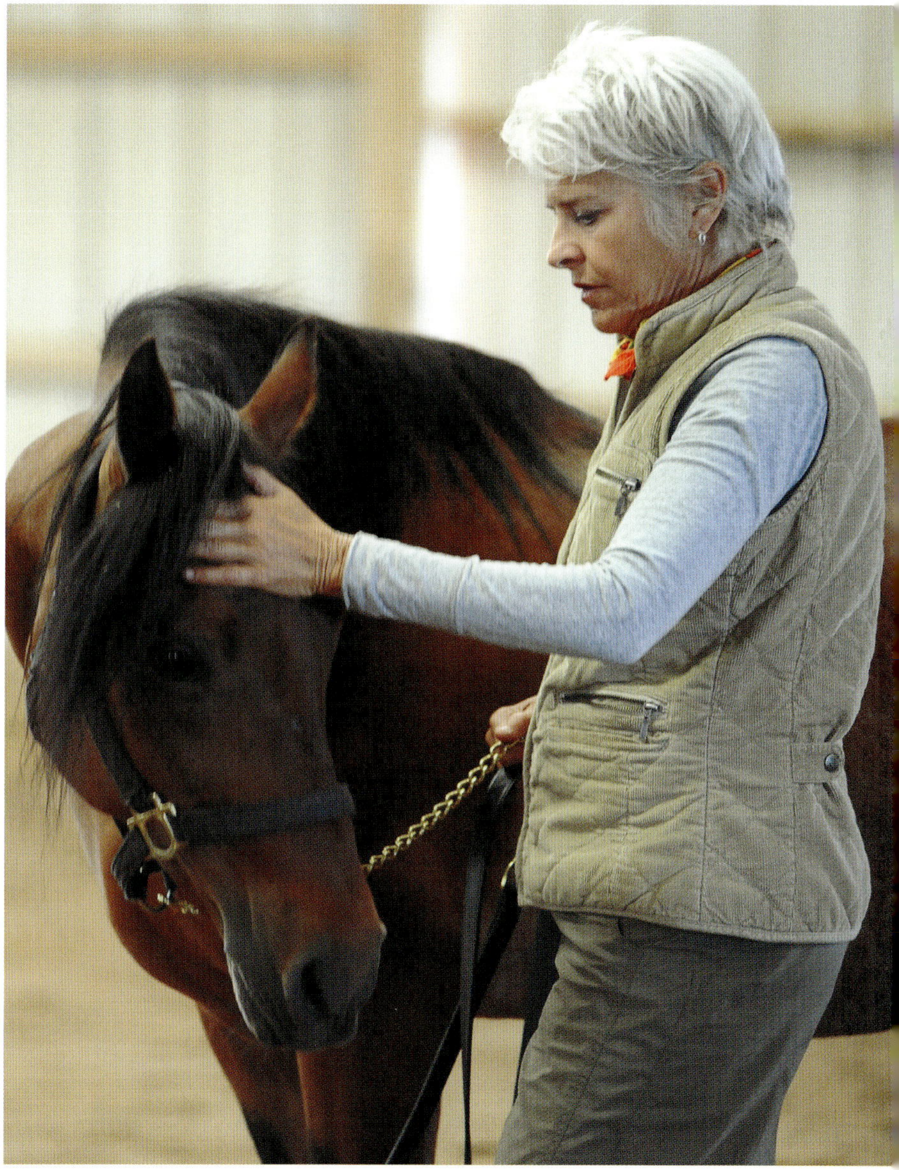

▲ **5.5** Samson lowers his head for a forehead release. This is a change you can offer frequently and it always benefits the horse.

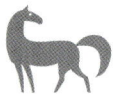

SEEING THE STILL POINT

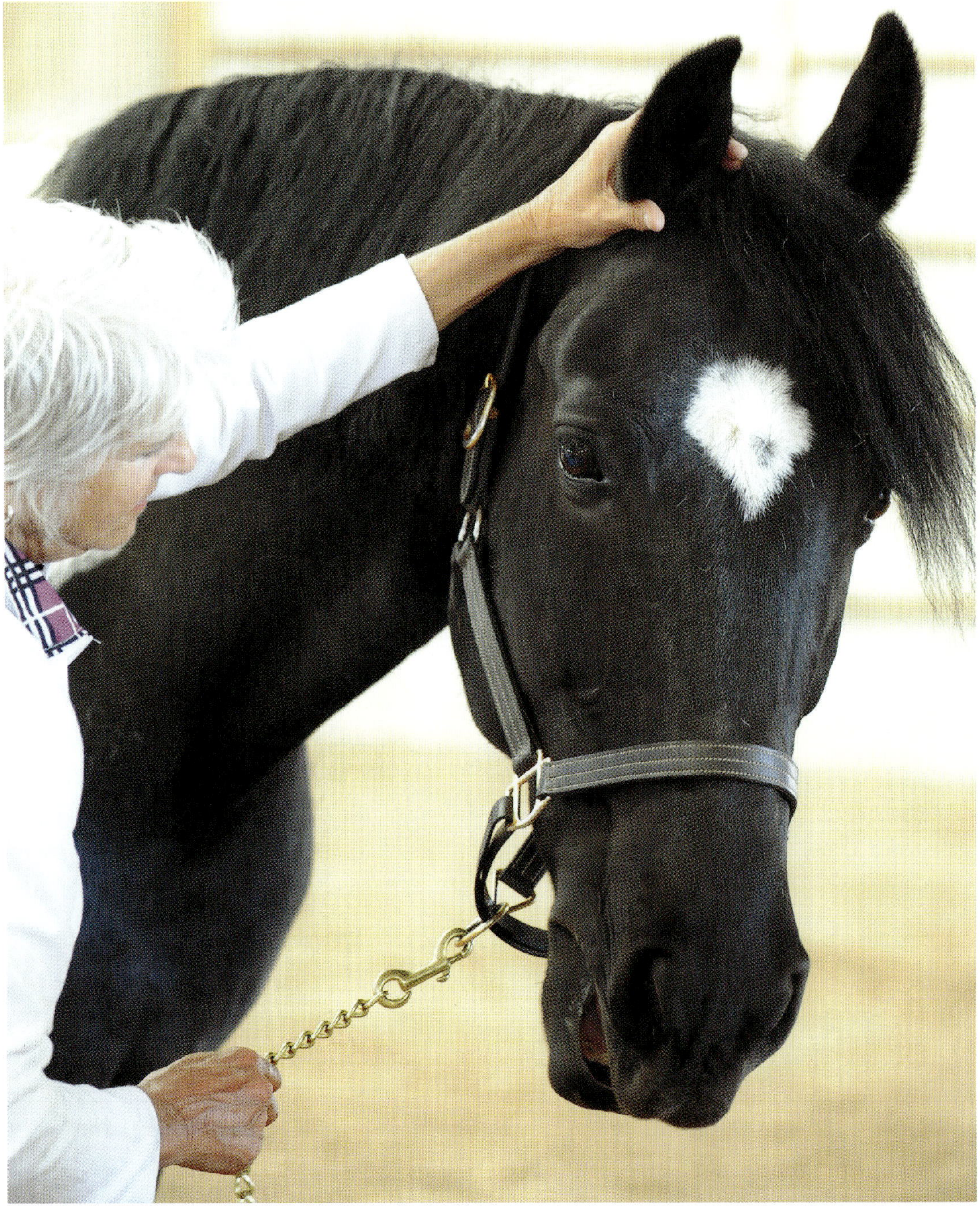

▶ **5.7** Beau models a Still Point experience here in an ear release.

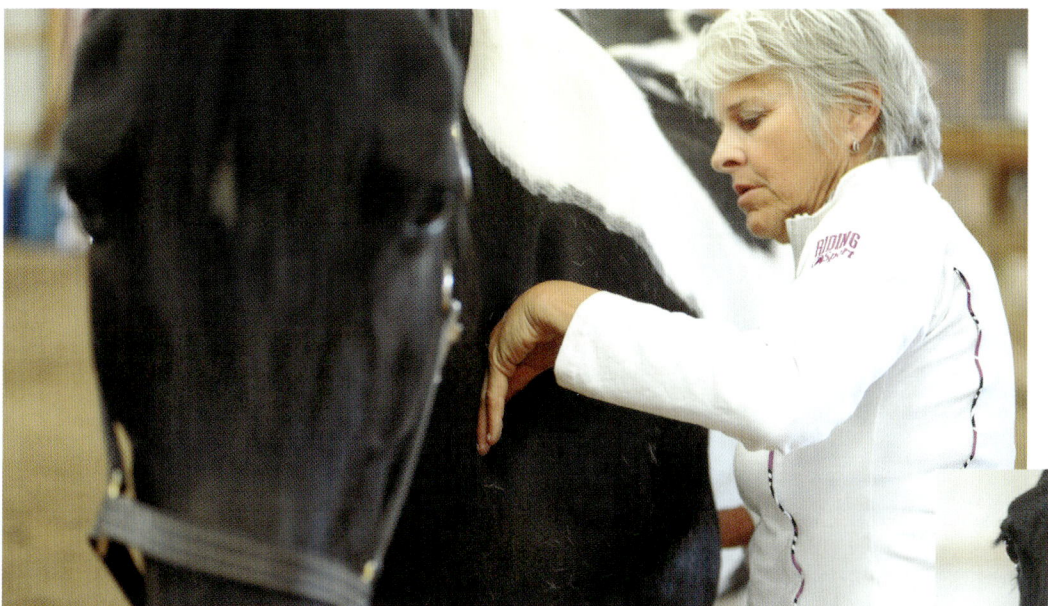

◀ **5.8** A shoulder crease change brings this Still Point for Beau.

▶ **5.9** Scout's in-mouth release brings a Still Point, despite his movement. I go with the movement, allowing the horse to find his way, and don't interrupt the change.

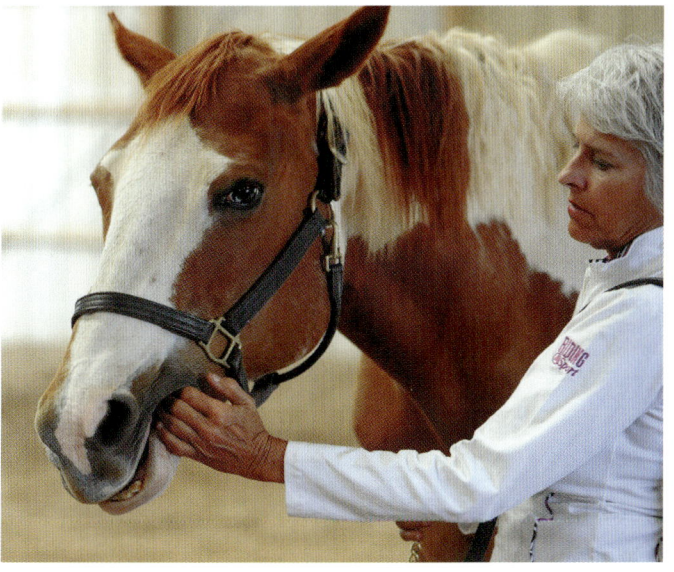

▲ **5.10** Jet's head change has a Still Point. Head releases often bring at least one Still Point. Always offer the horse a chance for more than one.

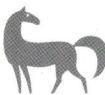

best offered frequently, perhaps three times weekly, at first. Horses crave this change when their head isn't balanced. Highly oral horses that cannot stand still without continually chewing on something always have an unbalanced head.

Mouth

When you look carefully at the horse's mouth, an imbalanced horse often shows a jutting or pouting lower lip that comes out past the upper lip. (Your inventory photos can remind you of where the horse started—see p. 34.) This gives the horse a clumsy looking mouth that usually changes with head balancing. The in-mouth, poll, and jaw releases transform the muzzle into a refined profile. This balancing normally takes about four sessions, depending on the horse. It can also happen in one session. Like a garden where growth seems sudden after months of slow progress, the horse suddenly looks very sensitive. His eye is soft and receptive, and he's much more cooperative. As the horse's lower jaw recedes, he has an attractive profile.

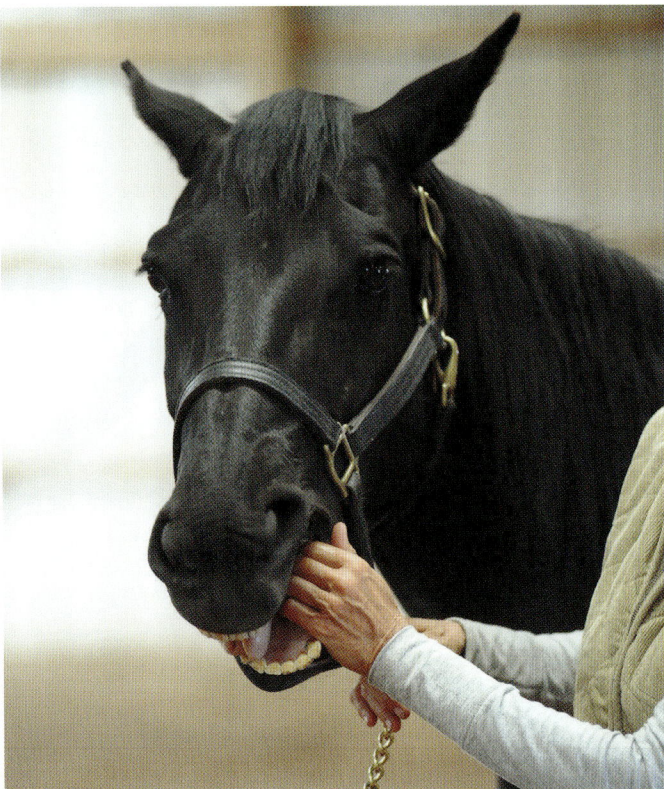

▲ **5.11** Jet works her mouth. It looks as if the horse will bite me but she is very careful of my hand.

INDICATIONS OF HEAD IMBALANCE

- High strung, anxious.

- Champing on or playing with the bit.

- Throwing the head up or side to side.

- Resistance to tacking up with the headstall.

- Resistance to leading.

- Resistance to wearing the halter.

- Poll stiffness under saddle.

- Twisting to one side under saddle (crookedness is often in the poll fascia).

- Cribbing.

- Unusually submissive herd behavior.

- Inability to eat well and keep weight on.

▶ **5.12** Remy works his front lip here. The web of my hand between my thumb and pointer finger leans up to the gum line in the horse's mouth. The horse applies the pressure that suits him. This is a very effective release to regularly offer the horse.

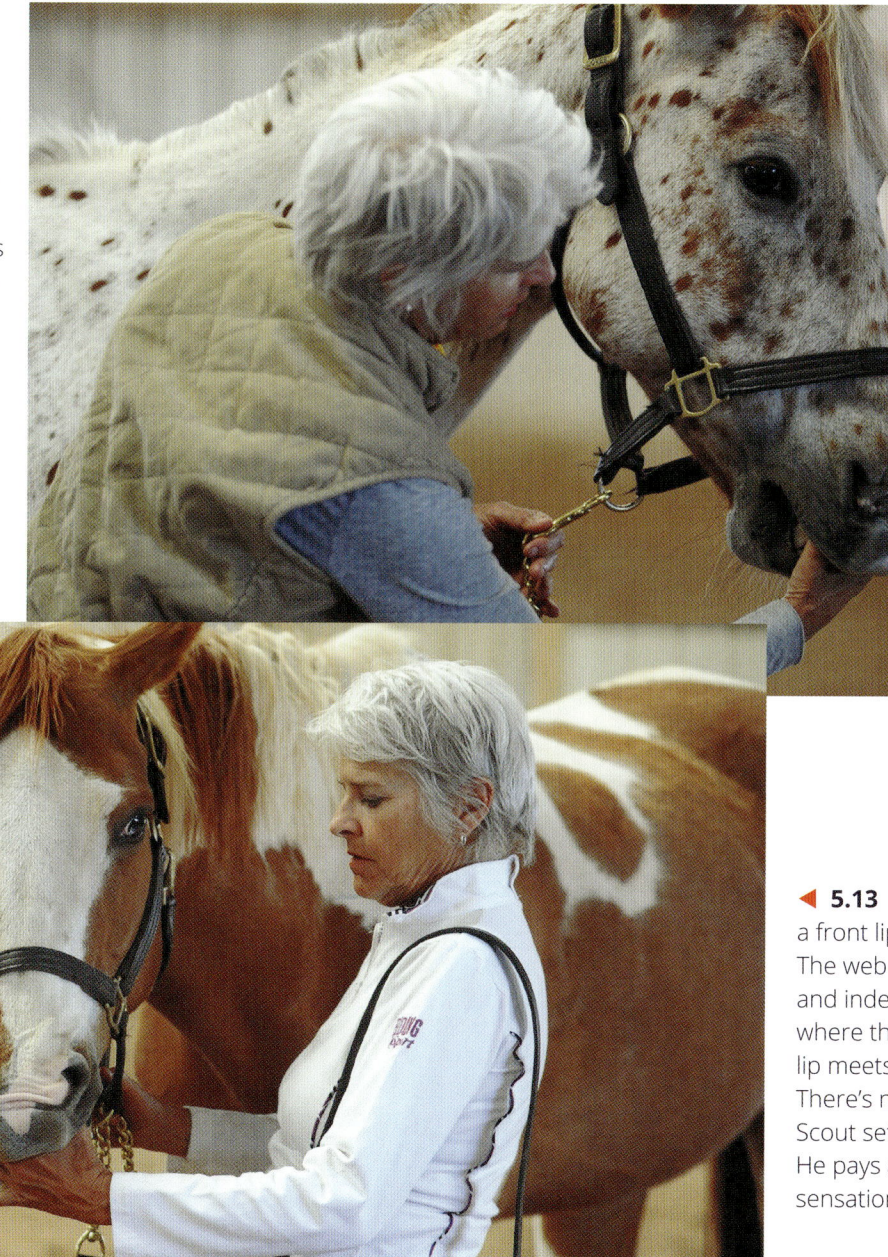

◀ **5.13** Scout enjoys a front lip release. The web of my thumb and index finger rests where the upper lip meets the gums. There's no pushing. I let Scout set the pressure. He pays attention to his sensations.

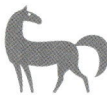

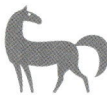

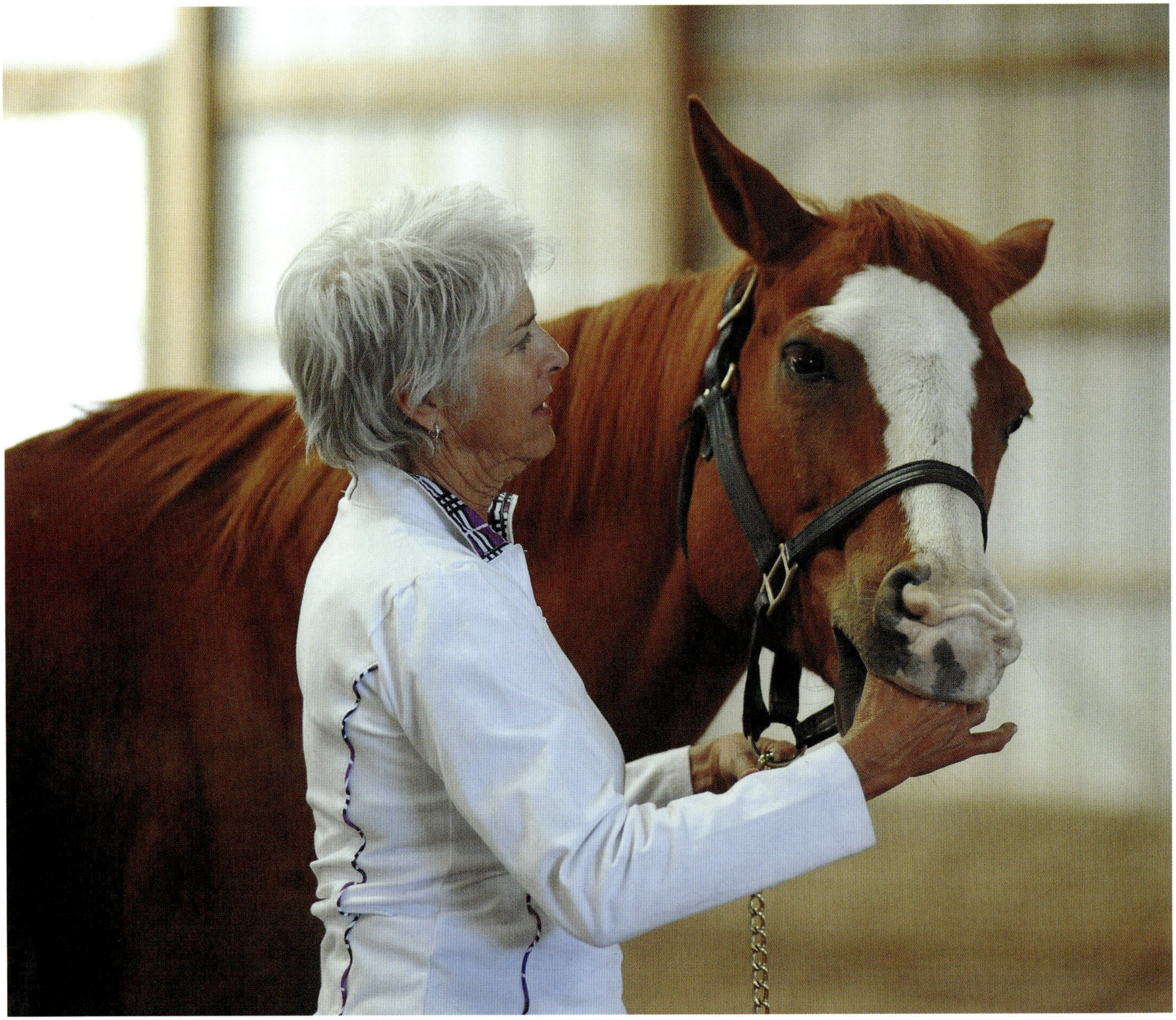

▲ **5.14** CT works his front lip in this mouth release. The horse flicks me away when he's finished.

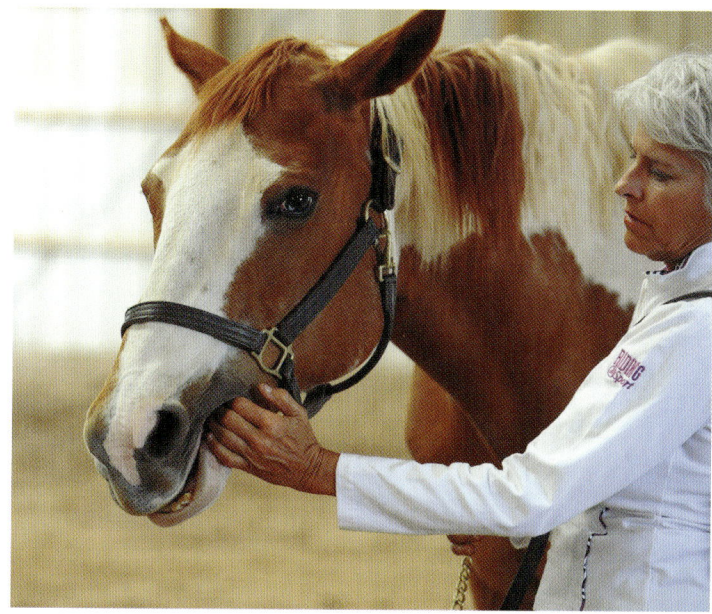

▲ **5.15** I slip my fingers into the space where the bit sits and just rest them there, without pushing. Scout does all the work, as I stimulate his movement. I offer this change on both sides. The horse usually prefers you to spend more time on his stiffer side.

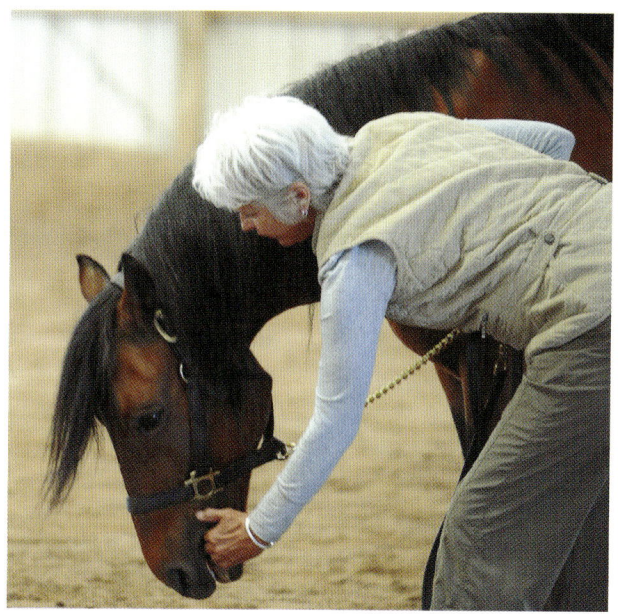

▲ **5.16** Samson lowers his head to work with the leverage he wants. I follow the horse's lead here for the best results.

When the horse will not permit in-mouth changes, it's often due to painful stiffness in the lips. To offer him a muzzle release, cup your hand on the upper lip and the lower with one soft hand at a time. There's no rush or pressure in your touch. Work in small sessions, as he cannot always absorb an entire change at once. You will be rewarded with a soft mouth and much less resistance to the bit. Once the very stiff muzzle has softened, it's easier for the horse to cooperate with in-mouth releases (fig. 5.13). If he doesn't like them, after your repeated attempts, don't worry. He may not need them. You can try them at another time.

Mouth Releases

Mouth releases are easy when the horse agrees. Using the web of skin between the thumb and index finger, slide your hand into the space between the horse's upper lip and gum, at the top (fig. 5.14). Rest your hand there without moving the fingers. The horse may sink his head into your hand to adjust the contact for the most gain once he knows what you are doing. Often, the horse will move his teeth and lips, actively participating with the release. Sometimes, the horse can throw his head up and down to get the contact he needs for complete change. His participation is vital to full change. When he moves his head down or up, follow that

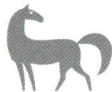

movement with the hand still in his mouth. He will flick you out when he's finished.

Side of Mouth Release

Rest two fingers on the bar of the horse's jaw where the bit rests (figs. 5.15 & 5.16). Don't massage. Let the

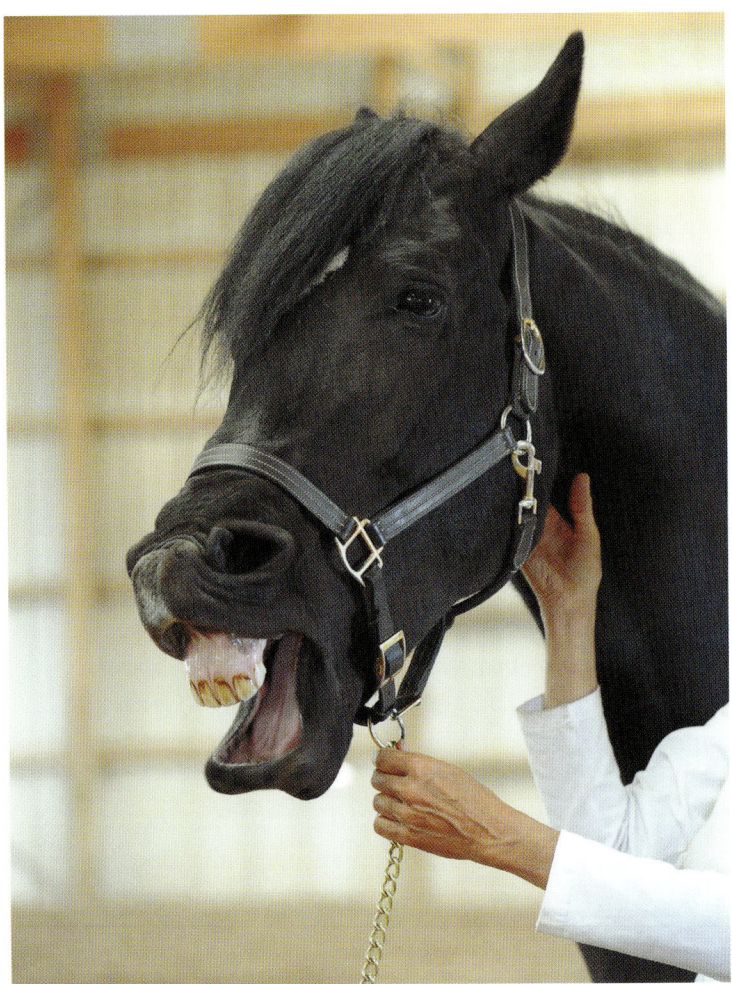

▲ **5.17** Beau yawns with relief.

fingers rest there without exerting pressure. The horse will move as needed to make the contact active for him. Repeat this release on each side of the head. It is very helpful for balancing the jaw and the cranium. Sometimes the horse needs to circle while you are working in his mouth. This actually improves the release for him, so follow him as long as you can do it safely. Gaited horses, especially, need to move while having head releases and changes. This release is excellent for regular balancing weekly or whenever you fit it in, either before or after a ride.

Eyes and Nostrils

Look carefully at the eyes and nostrils to notice if they're even. When an eye or nostril is farther up, that's imbalance. Maybe, it's rotated backward. Sometimes the eyes are not even, but the nostrils appear to be. These are all variations on imbalance that the horse may have had for years. Photos will help you see the reality of the horse's face. Don't worry about how the head looks; it changes rapidly and self-intelligently. Hands on the forehead, poll, jaw, and inside the mouth affect the changes as the horse approves and needs. When the horse no longer accepts contact, you know that he either needs a break to digest change, or that change is not needed.

Jaw

The jaw often reveals collection strain. Sometimes, a horse has an uneven jaw. Perhaps he has been turned hard and often in one direction. Perhaps his rider used one hand more severely. Or the heavy side compensated for the weaker side. Like humans, most horses

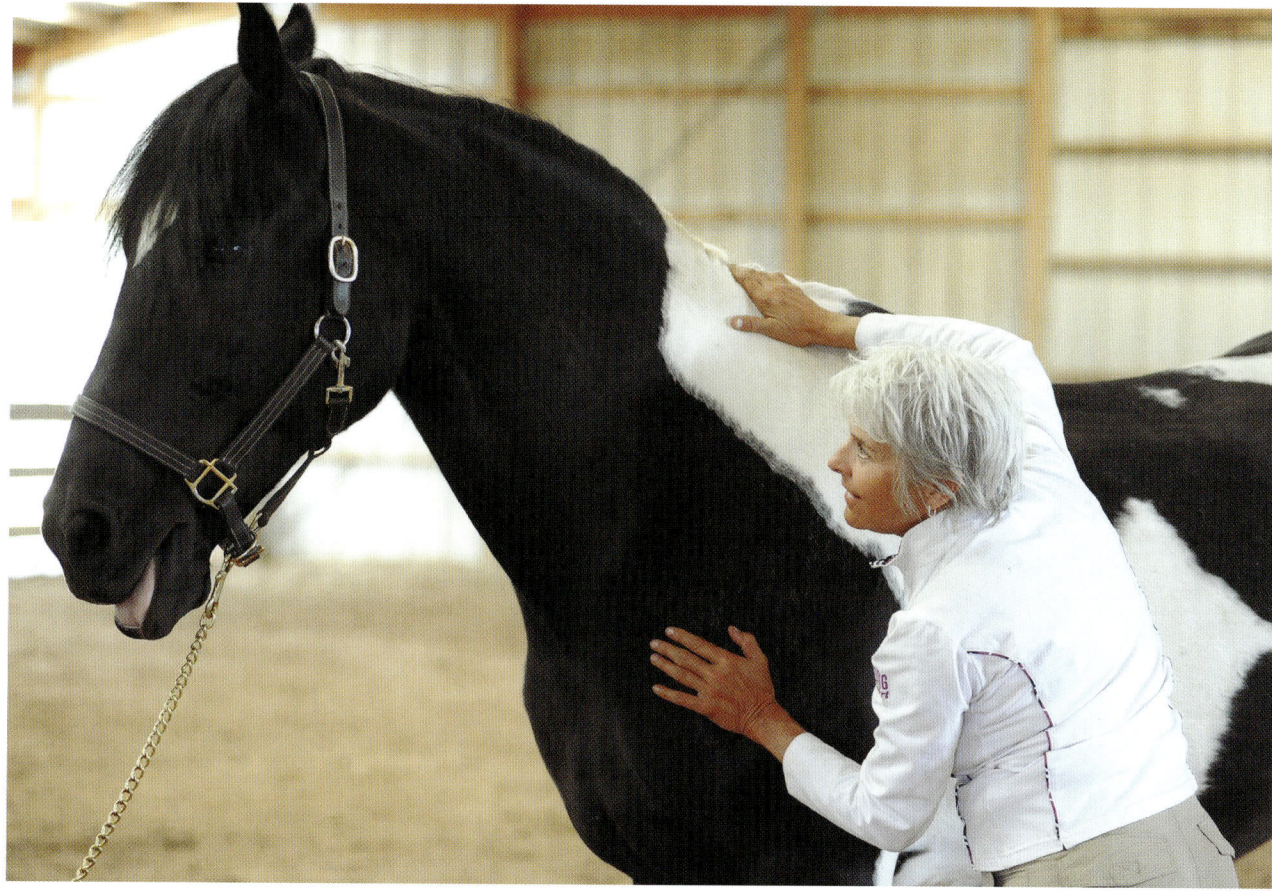

have one dominant side. Start by sinking your fingers gently upward, under the jaw, softly and slowly. Jaw balance also allows the horse's head to sit properly on his neck (fig. 5.17).

Shoulders

As I've discussed, the shoulder is the center of gravity for the horse. Shoulder tightness is often the source of

hind end lameness, collection problems, and an inability to take the correct lead. The shoulder muscle group is the only muscle group not attached directly to the skeleton. This gives the horse a huge advantage when running over rough country. His front legs can spring up and down easily without straining his skeleton's stability. The hind end, with its accordion bone structure, follows in perfect congruence and stability. A shoulder that can absorb terrain and speed changes is vital for a

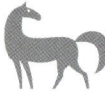

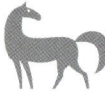

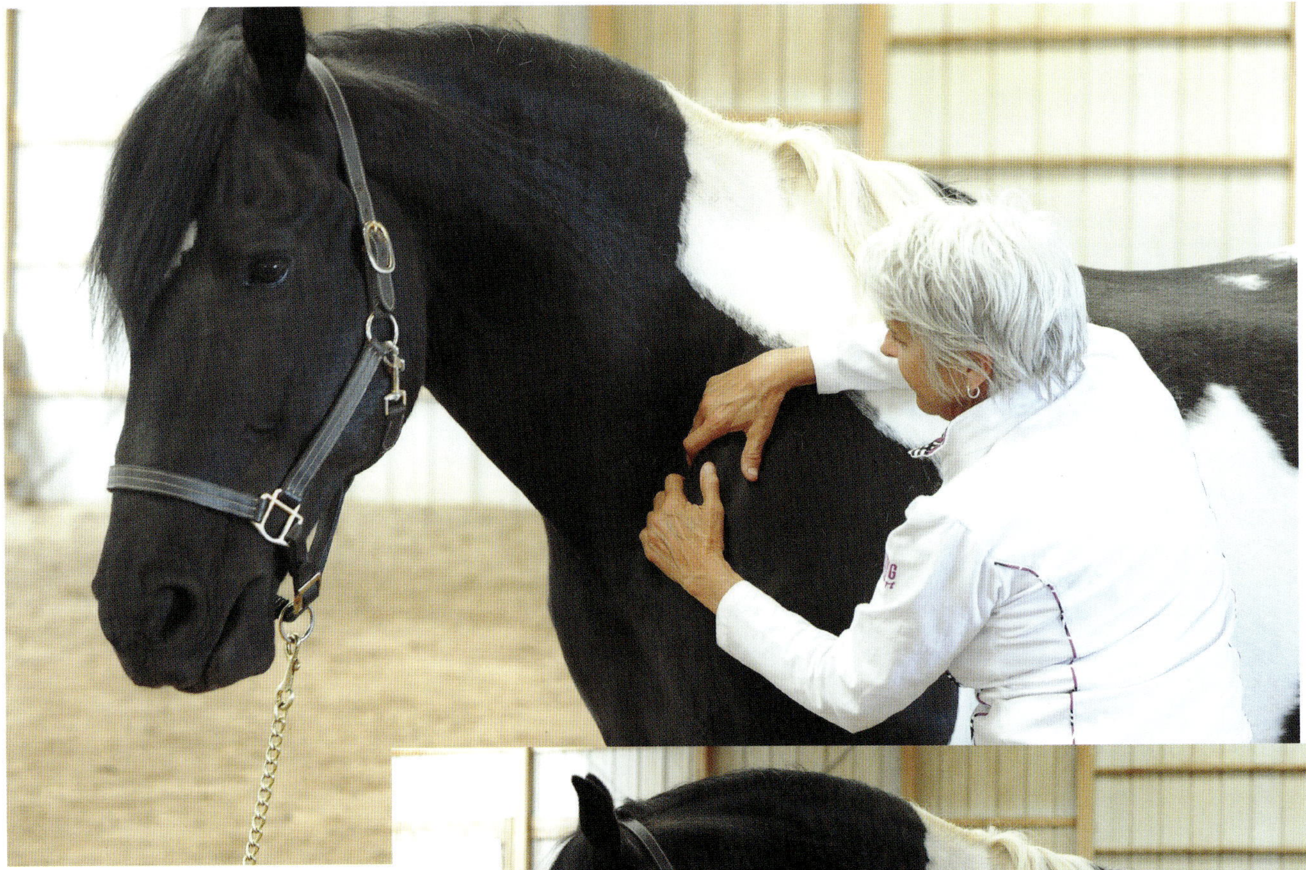

▲ **5.19** My fingers are in Beau's shoulder crease.

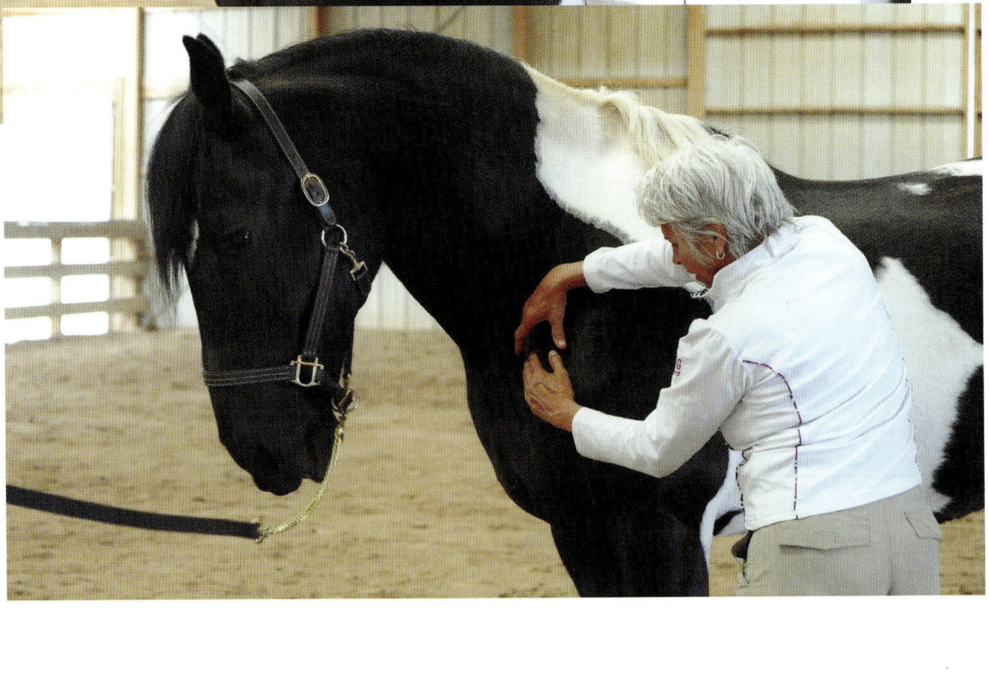

▶ **5.20** Beau arches his neck as he feels the space increase inside his shoulder.

running animal. A horse needs a freely moving shoulder structure to retain his gravity-center stability.

Many horses have stiff, wooden shoulders that create a nick in the withers. Your palm softens it without pain. For a stiff horse, use the palm release on the top of the withers, along the ridge of the neck, and over the entire shoulder area.

An improved topline rewards those who take the time to open the withers and neck-ridge fascia. In a horse with a light-looking or undeveloped front end, a tight shoulder crease is usually the cause. Amazingly, once you have opened the crease for the horse, it's easy to maintain. Keeping the shoulder creases open and supple truly releases the stride limits, as well as raising the withers.

How to Do a Shoulder Crease Release

To begin shoulder balancing, first stroke the muscles with the palms. Go in both directions, checking to see which is stiffer. Healthy tissue should have a flexible quality to it. It's easier for the horse if you choose the more fluid shoulder first (figs. 5.18–5.20).

Let the palms melt the surface tissue waiting for change. Stroke down from the top of the withers and neck, using slow strokes. Continue this, working on both sides of the horse, until the tissue has softened and the horse is accepting of the fingers sliding inside the crease. As the fingers warm the fascia, the crease will open farther, and let the hand drop in progressively deeper. As the opening softens and fully opens, the hand slides inside all the way down the crease opening toward the chest. The fully opened shoulder crease allows the full fist, held softly, inside.

Patience and gradual work succeed in opening a shoulder crease. Practice with the horse in small sessions, spread over days. Horses are happy in this change if you are gentle with them. Usually, it only takes a few sessions to open the crease completely. Once opened fully, a shoulder crease only needs occasional attention.

Withers

The withers are an area for regular checking (fig. 5.21). While the top of the withers seems to be mostly bone, you cap the withers with your palms to create heat for the fascia change. The changes spread up the neck and down into the shoulder.

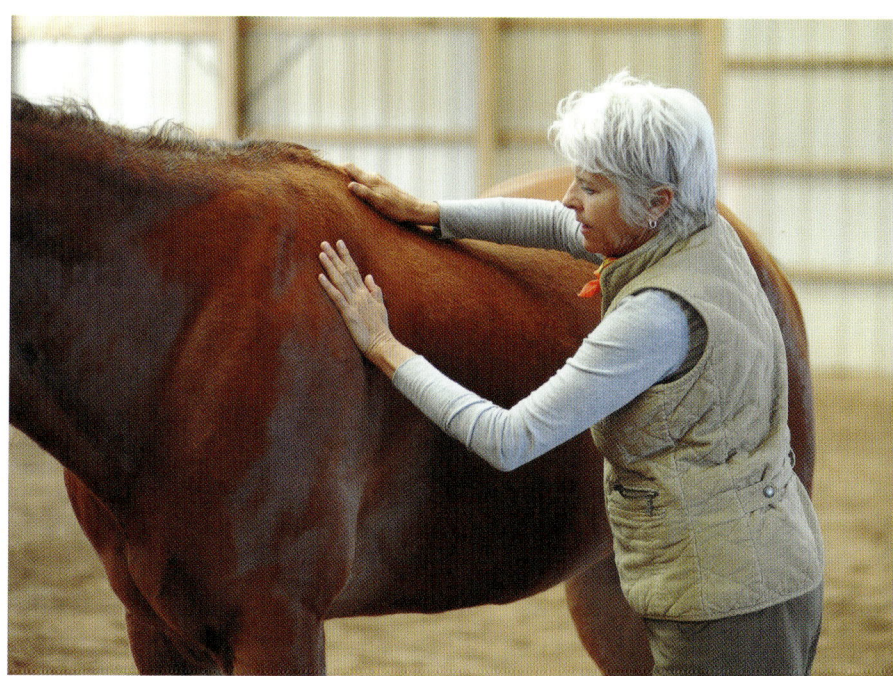

▲ **5.21** My palms soften stiff withers and shoulder fascia on EZ.

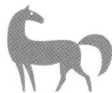

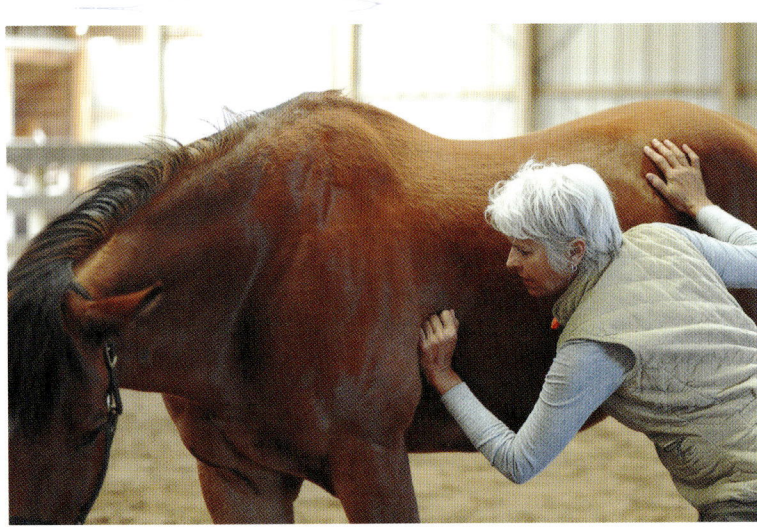

▲ **5.22** A slow, soft fist works well for a girth stroke. This is an area of strain.

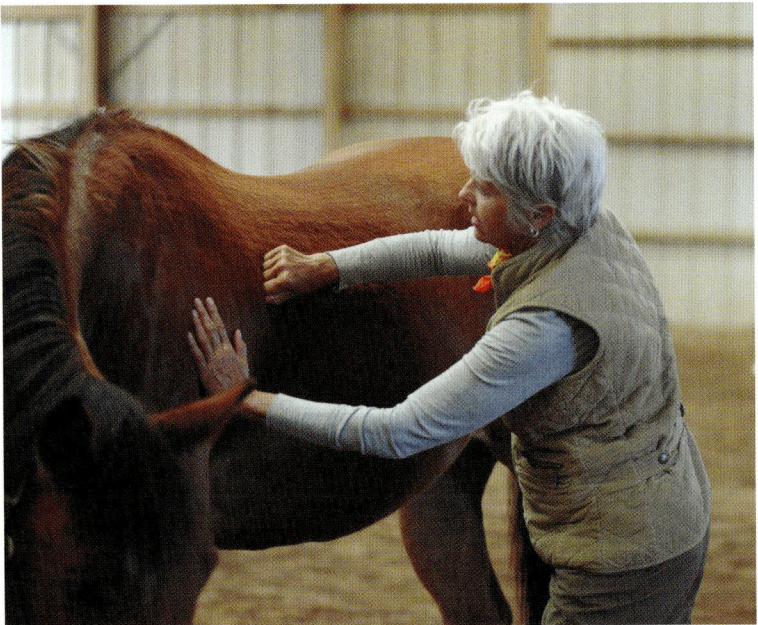

▲ **5.23** EZ curves his neck in as I do a barrel stroke. As the front and back ends of the horse begin to balance, the barrel responds quickly.

Release of the withers is extremely helpful for saddle-fit problems. One reason for saddle fit problems is that the horse's back is so compensated that he can't carry the saddle in a balanced way. Custom saddles don't resolve the problems from compensations in the withers, shoulders, and back; the fascia continues to tighten further, always changing the fit.

Barrel

As the shoulders and withers are balancing, be sure to work the barrel also so that it keeps up with the changes. You use a soft fist to stroke along the barrel horizontally, making three or four rows of stroke. Then, you use your fingers to stroke down the intercostal fascia between each rib. There are 18 ribs, so that means nine strokes downward between the ribs. Then use the soft fist again to go up vertically starting at the girth area, making about four strokes across the entire barrel.

Use the flat palm on areas of clumping or sensitivity, such as the posterior abdominal area. Always proceed slowly and carefully in the girth area (figs. 5.22 & 5.23). Many horses are tight and stiff here and will negatively react to a rapid or rough approach in the girth area.

Hindquarters

The hindquarters require maintenance balancing, as well. The stroke-pattern diagrams in chapter 4 show different stroke pattern options for the hindquarters (see p. 61). The hip point deserves your special focus (fig. 5.24). To open the fascia on the hip point, you work around it with your palms, including cupping it to melt the tightness. This is a high strain area for nearly all horses.

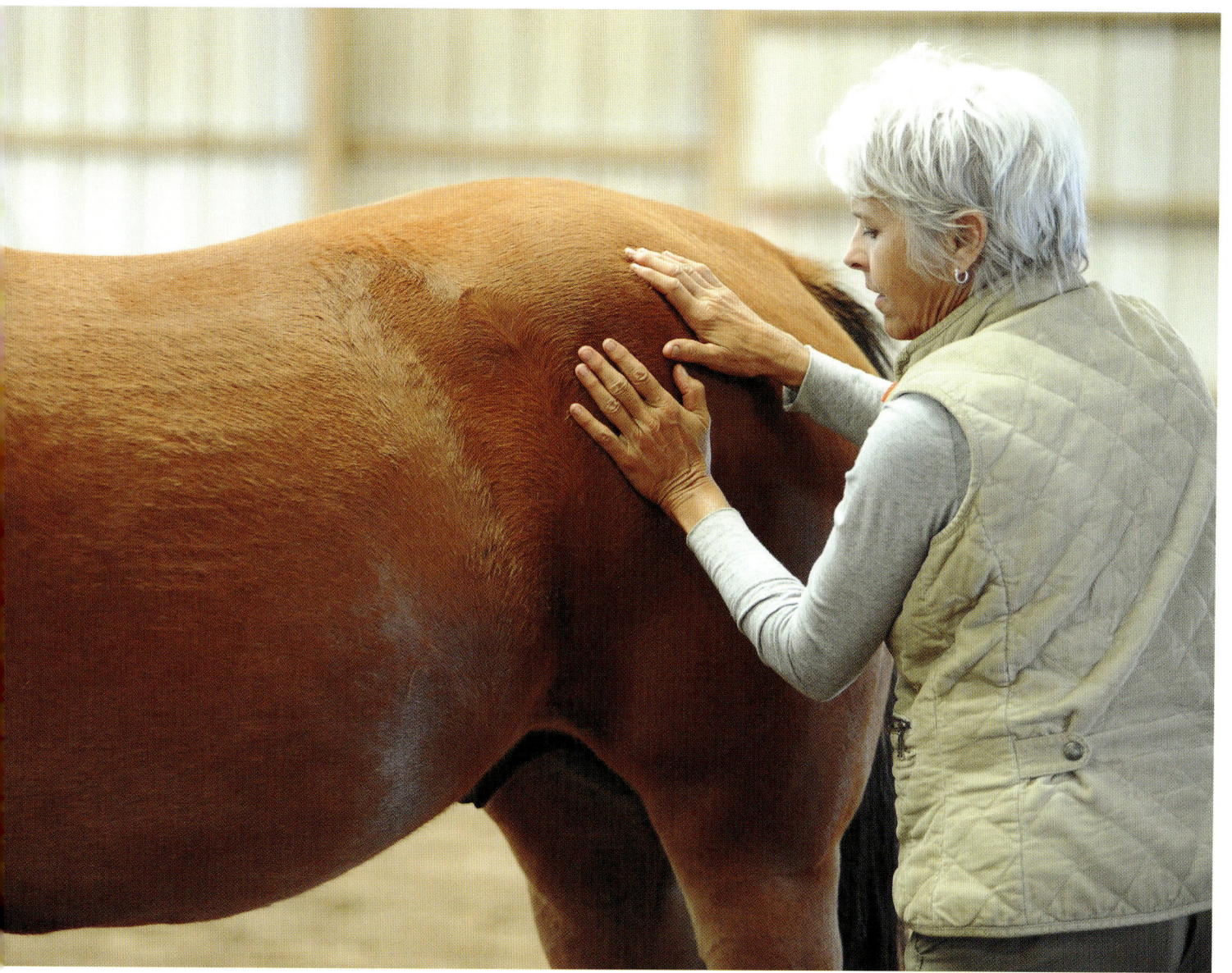

▲ **5.24** I work around EZ's hip point with my palms. This area limits pelvic movements when it's tight and compensated.

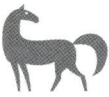

COMMON CONFORMATION BALANCING QUESTIONS AND ANSWERS

Do horses get "sore" with fascia changes?

If the hands are not pushing, the horse does not feel any pain or soreness after sessions. A very stiff horse—or a horse with a chronic injury history—definitely requires time to "organize" before returning to regular activity. The extremely tight horse may look "wobbly" after the session due to the new space throughout his body. He needs a few days being turned out to organize his body again.

How do I return my horse to work after a long rest?

To return a horse to active work after years or months of stiffness and disability, the walk is the best exercise. I discuss this in chapter 7 (see p. 115). The horse balances his entire hindquarters again, reintegrates his sacral juncture and finds his center of gravity—the shoulders—through walking. Stops, or halts, serve to help the horse "find" his sacral juncture again, since it often was numbed by the compression of many months or even years. The horse finds his range of motion by walking straight or in gentle curves. Small circles or round pens are not appropriate exercise until the horse has rebalanced laterally.

My trainer thinks the horse needs to work more; why can't we return to our lessons?

When restoring a horse to full ability after an extended loss of movement or an injury, the usual work routine is not appropriate. The horse can't do his former work well until he is organized and integrated again. It's best to take the same approach that humans take in rehabilitation after a surgery or accident: careful, regular, and quite moderate exercise. Former training or competition goals should wait until the horse shows ability to perform at those levels consistently.

The croup is another area where flat hands work very well for fascia changes. It is very dense and usually stiff, like the sacral juncture. It melts with patience, and it deserves your regular attention. Visually, lumps and other variations show the stress of the vertebrae, especially fast stops, jumps, and collection work.

What to Do After Scanning and Balancing Sessions

You can help your horse assimilate his changes more fully by giving him a little time off and turnout. He integrates himself and organizes more quickly and completely when this happens, thus progressing the changes better than if he returns to standing still in a stall or heads right in to a lesson. He often remains in Still Point for some time, digesting his changes. He seems relaxed and energized. It's tempting to ride immediately after and test out the changes, but when you wait a day or two, it rewards you both.

If you do ride after a session, it's best to warm up slowly. Walking at least 20 minutes is a good start. Transitions should not be rushed. Tight circles or demanding collection exercises will hinder your horse's integration of the new tissue connections. You will both benefit from easing into complex work over a week's time.

Grayson: Follow the Cues

Savannah's horse's first session showed her how to follow him, regardless of her own agenda. She found her large Hanoverian gelding "Grayson" unfocused. He threw his head continually; he wasn't easy to handle despite careful training. She contacted me.

After I had done a scan on Grayson, he didn't settle into the hand contact or strokes. He circled continually. Immediately, I slipped my hand into the side of his mouth. That was what he wanted. The entire session ended up being 50 minutes of head balancing in the mouth, poll, and jaw.

This session is an excellent example of how following the horse's cues can bring success. No matter how you intend to organize your bodywork session, the horse often prioritizes your contact. By agreeing with what the horse tells you he needs, you have his approval and can help him.

Savannah was very pleased with her horse's new ability to focus, resulting from one Conformation Balancing session.

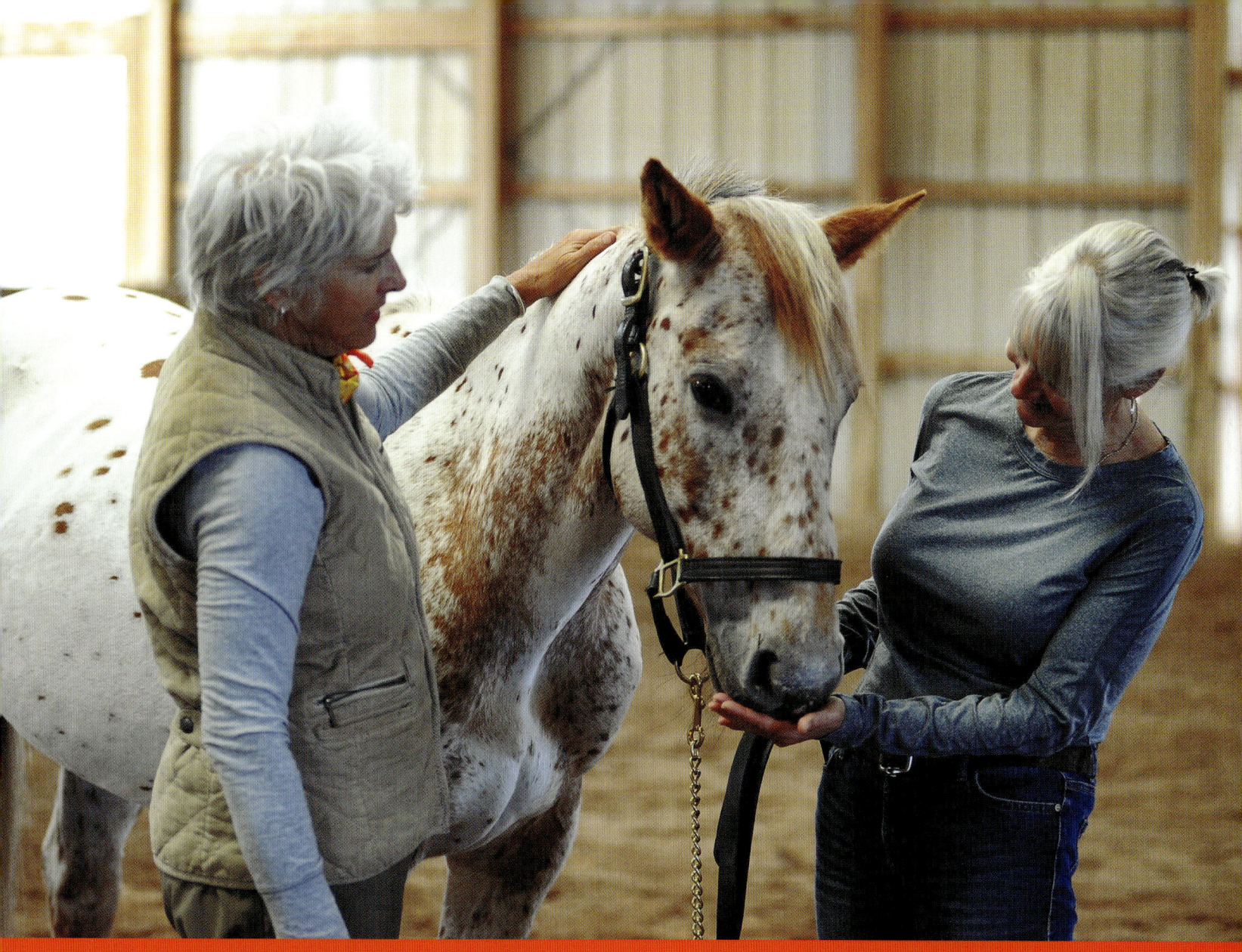

6 | Problem-Solving

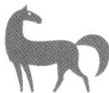

Resolving Issues with Conformation Balancing

Let's discuss some difficult situations that are resolved by Conformation Balancing. Chronically unbalanced horses are often "accident-prone" and get injured more than a balanced, fit horse. Although a horse may make progress, when there are still imbalances, some "old stuff" returns, eventually.

Meanwhile, the relapses happen in various ways. Accidents and injuries can be widely varied and seem very unrelated—unless you connect the dots. With continual balancing work, breakthroughs occur to clear the jam-up of stuck tissue.

As major areas become free of compensations and imbalance, the horse shows a new athletic ability to move well and avoid accidents. With increased consciousness, the horse makes fewer "mistakes" and shows better judgment. He is seldom injured. He doesn't panic often, but if he does, he stops and waits for clarity. Horses actually progress beyond instincts, just as humans do.

Stumbling

Stumbling results from imbalance; it is often resolved by attentive work on the knees and shoulders. One knee is often the source of the problem (figs. 6.1 & 6.2). Use your hands sensitively to find the tight, compensating tissue, by moving up and down the leg. It is often on

> Problems often start "higher" on the horse. First, look for imbalance in the shoulders and sacral/loin area before assuming the knees or stifles are the problem.

the medial (inside) part of the knee, but all areas of the knee should be addressed, including above and below it. Follow the sensations down the leg to the fetlock, and up the leg to the elbow, as well, searching for the entire area affected.

The horse responds when you have found the key area of strain. He will usually sigh, breathe out, or half close his eyes as "approval cues" that the hands have found the spot. This area deserves repeated releases. It's good to make notes about which knee, and the date of the work, for your records. Also check the other knee and the opposite shoulder.

The fetlock, pastern, and coronet band are also included in your hand contact. As always, attention to hoof care is part of the overview in any tripping habits, as well as a veterinary diagnosis ruling out causes unrelated to fascia balancing.

The Fragile Stifle

The stifle is perhaps the most sensitive part of the accordion-like structure of the horse's hindquarters. The stifle responds well to flat palm contact and is resilient in its potential for recovery from strain. You can help with careful, soft palm changes that allow the entire hindquarters area to reorganize.

In this area, most of all, you must proceed at the horse's pace. He will not tolerate insensitive contact, and you work the entire hindquarters and tail equally when restoring a stifle. Always use a palm here, never

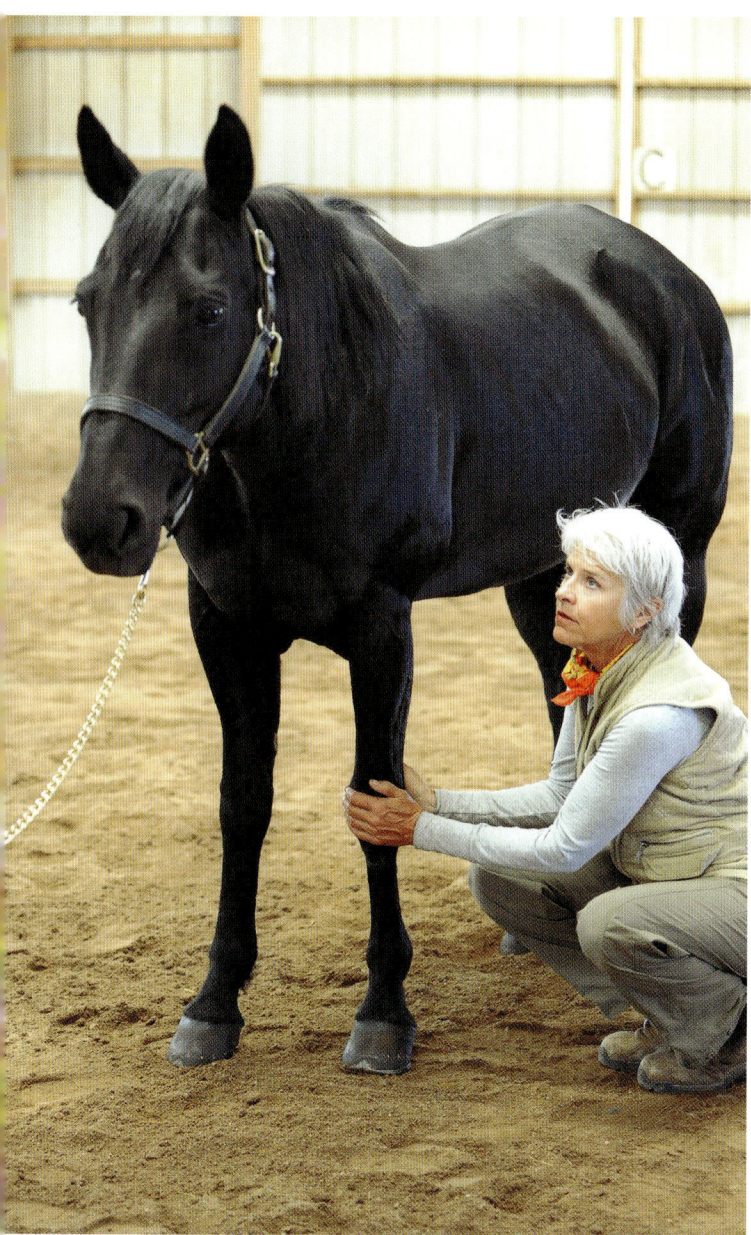

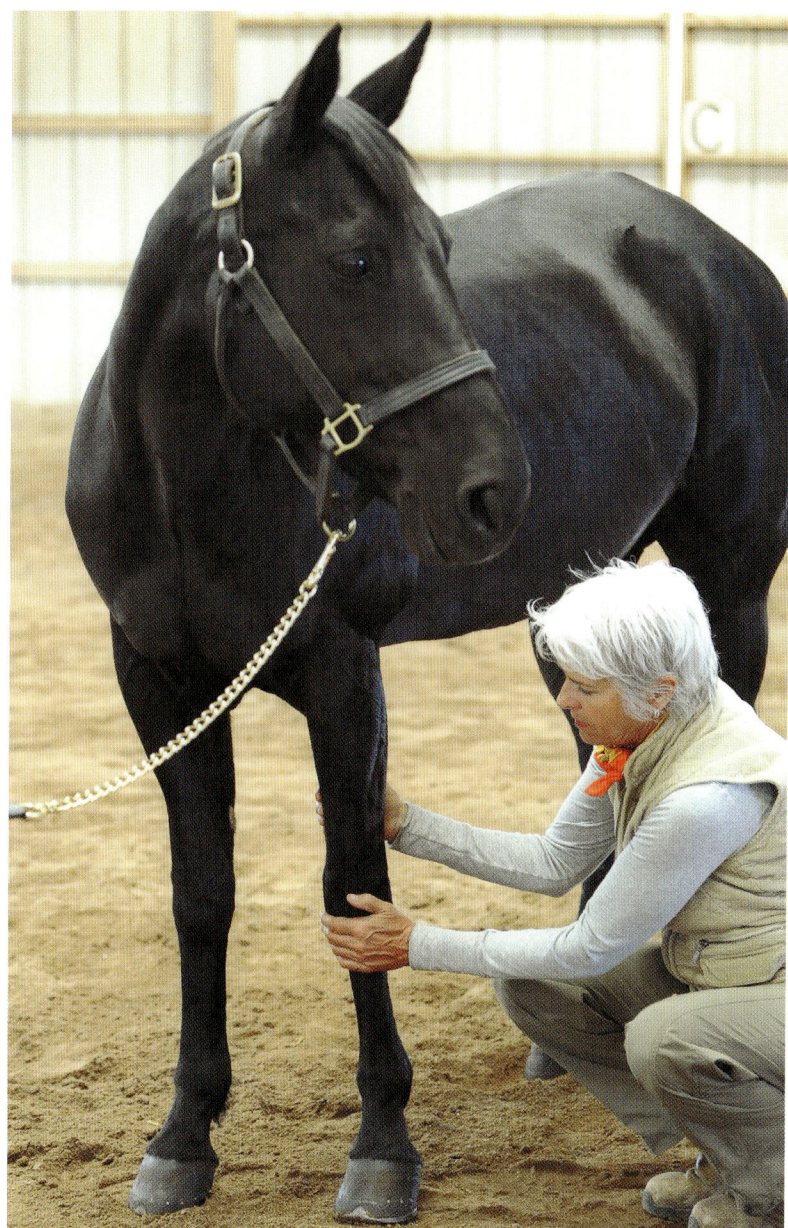

▲ **6.1** Jet has a Still Point as I cup her knee in my hands to release knee fascia. I wait to feel the strain surface; this is a common area of strain.

▲ **6.2** Jet attentively stands still as I continue wrapping my hands up her foreleg to release her knee strain.

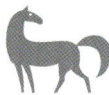

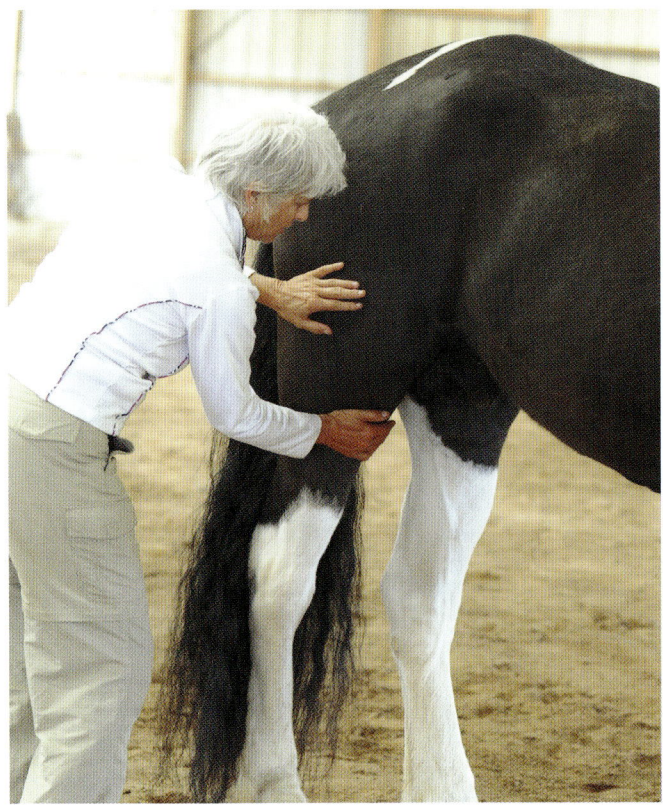

▲ **6.3** Beau accepts stifle change easily. Some horses find this contact stressful and guard themselves.

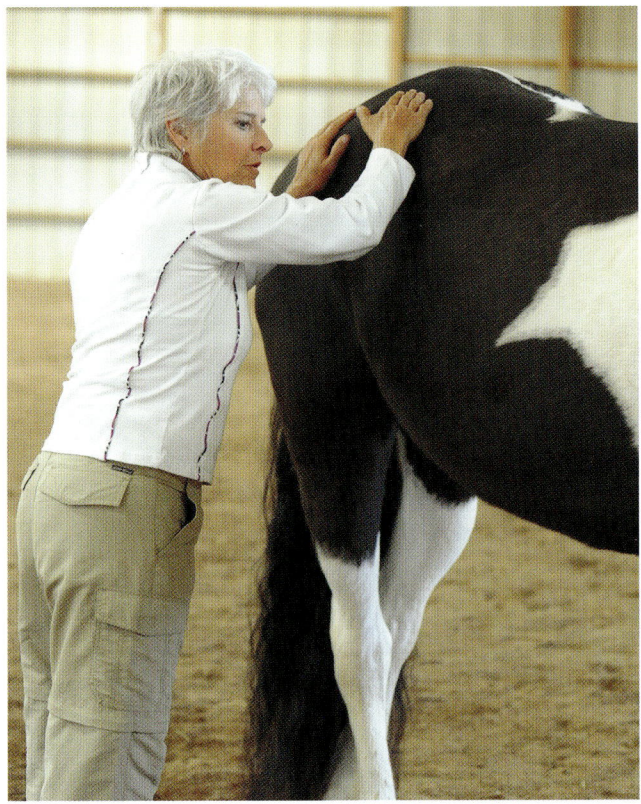

▲ **6.4** Notice the stance of Beau's rear legs; this is an "offset" stance and is showing sacral/pelvic imbalance.

a fist or knuckle. This is a key predator-attack area for horses, and their response to unacceptable contact is immediate (figs. 6.3 & 6.4).

Pullback Injuries

Horses are often tied to posts or fences; a pullback accident is when things go wrong and the horse pulls back hard, or rears up and pulls back, creating a huge torque on his poll and head. Additionally it causes neck, shoulders, withers, and barrel strain. It is a high impact accident, and it can last a horse's entire life.

The fascia effects are deep. When the horse can accept contact, use a palm, letting hand heat do the change. It will not be comfortable for the horse to experience any stretching or pulling. Palm contact effects the desired changes. Repeat the contact often and respect the horse's limits. The emotional trauma release is vital here; stay with the contact, without interruption. When the fascial tissue has been fully released, the trauma is usually gone, as well. Poll, in-mouth releases, and jaw changes should be where you begin. Then, open shoulder creases, "melt" the stuck withers, and open the elbows until they are wide. Pectorals also benefit from palm strokes. After the front end, address the sacral/loin juncture, then the dock and tail. This work should be repeated until the horse moves well consistently. If the horse doesn't tie well, a pullback accident is likely in his history. The mental change for the horse is usually prompt. The horse will accept being tied easily when all the balancing change is complete (figs. 6.5–6.7).

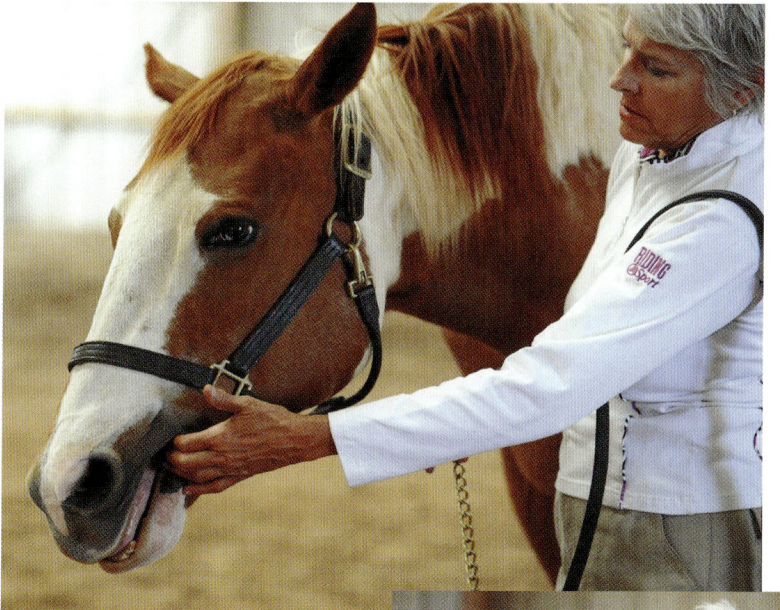

▲ **6.5** Scout enjoys an in-mouth release. The benefits of this change are impossible to overestimate, due to bitting effects, pullback incidents, and other head-related stress.

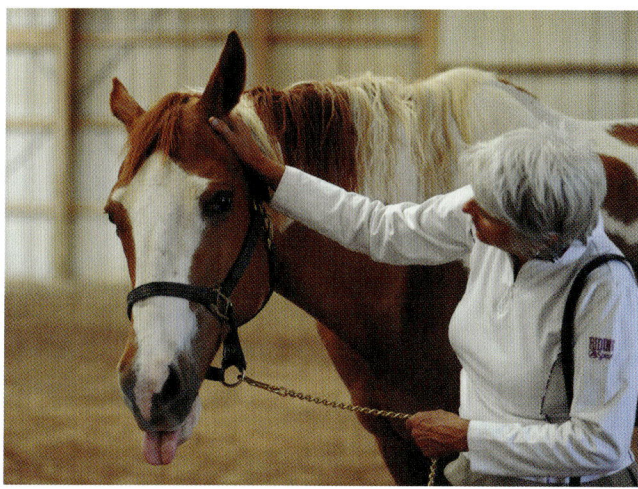

▲ **6.6** Ear releases are part of any head change, including those following pullback incidents. Scout enjoys this change.

◀ **6.7** Remy intently feels the change as his ear fascia balances. Ear changes often transform an anxious horse into a calm, poised one. As noted, be sure tack doesn't pinch the base of the ear.

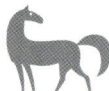

General Accident in Front or Behind

When the horse has begun to heal from an accident, remember his body is now compensating in thousands of ways. If it was a hind injury, you should be especially aware of shoulder and neck fascia strain, and the poll also. The barrel hides strain from a hind injury or strain.

When the accident is in front, pay close attention to the poll, tail, and sacral area as compensating parts. If it's a new horse, or a horse with undisclosed history, notice behaviors indicating problem areas; these can include inconsistencies, guarding, and fear. An accident leaves a cellular record that training doesn't address. The clues are usually in the horse's behavior.

A horse kicked in the ilium or hindquarters often shows a "dent." It's a common area for this kind of rough social behavior. The kick also unbalances the head, resulting in uneven eyes and nostrils. Head and poll balance returns quickly with repeated poll releases and in-mouth work. The forehead also needs flat palm releases, perhaps many times for full resolution, as well as ear changes. With patience, this entire problem can be balanced, instead of losing a good horse. Be sure to include tail changes, as they are probably much needed. Kicks look dramatic and deep, but tissue responds well to consistent fascial balancing.

Patrick: A Horse Restored

Patrick, a handsome Appendix Quarter Horse gelding, had been in a very difficult pasture situation where he was bullied and experienced injuries that ruined his fitness and caused him to lose a lot of weight. His owner moved him as fast as she could and did an extensive vet check. His uneven head created an offset jaw so that even dental work didn't help him eat well enough to gain the weight he needed. He was a mass of imbalances: front and back and side to side.

We worked with him regularly, focusing on his jaw, head, poll, and mouth so he could eat better. Then we opened his shoulder creases and adductors. His broomstick tail was another major focus. The barrel came next, and the elbows, too. A year later with six sessions, he looked nearly normal. Two years later, he was in show condition and stabilized. His happy owner rides the rugged mountains with ease, and Patrick is happily pastured with a compatible mare.

The Sacral Juncture

The sacral juncture is where the pelvis connects to the back (spine). This lower-back area is an important area of stability and it is a crucial area on the horse. This juncture takes even more strain when the head is unbalanced since strain passes along each vertebra, sharing the load, all the way to the last joint of the tail.

All training practices and riding disciplines require hind flexion and pelvic ease of movement. So, this is an area of high stress, no matter what the riding discipline. The sacral juncture is often so tight that it feels wooden and numb—this hurts the horse. If this area is hard and wood-like, there are adhesions taking care of the strain. But the adhesions also limit the flexibility.

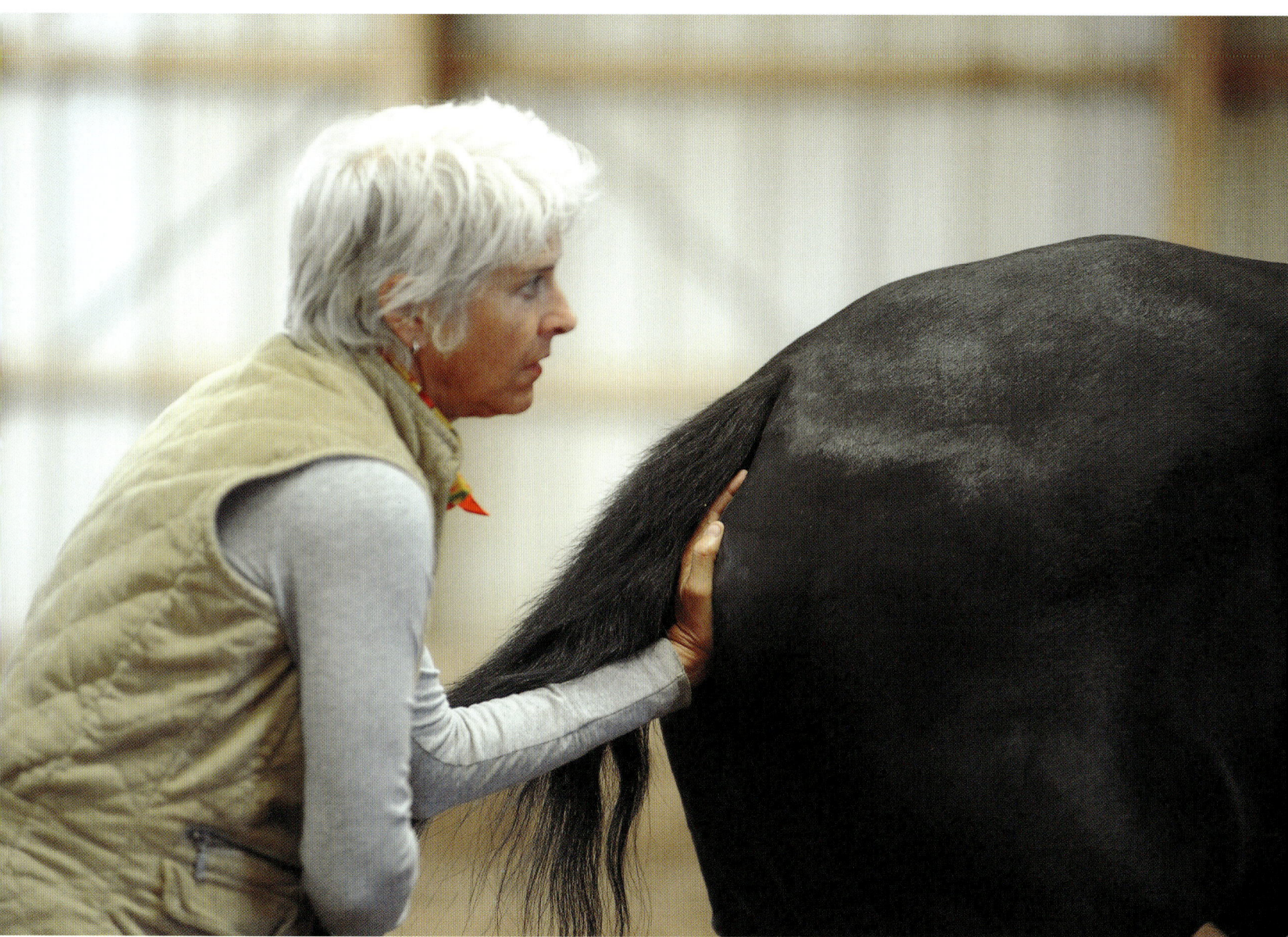

▲ **6.8** Jet models the ilium change here. I lean into the tissue, not pushing. I'm working just above the ilium, or seat bone. This is a common area for horses to kick each other. The muscle will often show a dent, which can disappear.

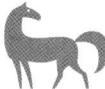

Clues to Sacral Strain

- Resistance to collection, revealing pain.

- Problems at the canter; also a sign of pain.

- Bucking or crowhopping (his back hurts).

- Raised vertebrae, indicating strain and imbalance.

- Sore back issues and saddle fit problems.

- A tight, rigid tail, indicating sacral tightness and compression.

The sacral juncture is a maintenance area. You should check it weekly and melt the hardness regularly with warm palms. It is often stiff, even on horses with no other complaints or issues. It is a common stress area for jumping and dressage horses. Even a young horse can look bony and "broken-backed" in the sacral area. This is a priority area for every session. You may stand for long minutes while your hands melt this very dense part of the horse with many compensations. It's worth the time!

The hindquarters can weigh 500 pounds. When the sacral juncture shows a dip or a "separation," the fascia is highly compensated. This area rewards all efforts. After you soften it using a flat palm, use a gentle twisting motion with both soft palms to help the fascia regain movement in all directions (see p. 63). Repeat this often for as long as it takes for the fascia to balance itself.

Tail releases are extremely helpful in changing the sacral-juncture area. Often, the horse has a very stiff or kinked tail. Hold the tail in your palms for the fascial change, as noted in the tail section of chapter 4 (see p. 75). The body has its own timing. Keep offering the change and improvements will come. This may require a few months due to the density of the area, but the sacral area does respond and the changes last. It's important to mention here that if the horse has a sacral strain, he should not be jumped or worked hard in collection.

Scars

Scars reveal accidents. Palm contact around the edges of a scar allows the edge fascia to spread farther. If the scar is old, it's often a mass of hardened adhesions, but it responds to your hand's heat promptly. Often, there is a lumpy tissue near scars, or an area that has thickened. Repeat warm contact over the area often, waiting minutes as old stuck fascia melts and opens to balance. Check the entire area, and, as always, look for diagonal compensation patterns on the other side of the horse for further adhesions from the old accident.

Gelding Scar Release

The gelding scar is often overlooked. When a horse is gelded, he may not heal evenly. His body may produce stiff adhesions in his groin that later impede collection or canter leads. You can use a warm, soft hand to hold the folds where the testicles once were. Cool, cold, or stuck tissue reveals an unbalanced healing, with many compensations for the horse. Softly and patiently, your warm hands can melt the stuck fascia (fig. 6.9). The gelding scar resumes normal temperature as it regains its fascial balance. Offer this more than once until the fascia feels completely normal and the tissue moves freely without restriction. This fascia change makes a huge difference especially in horses working in collection.

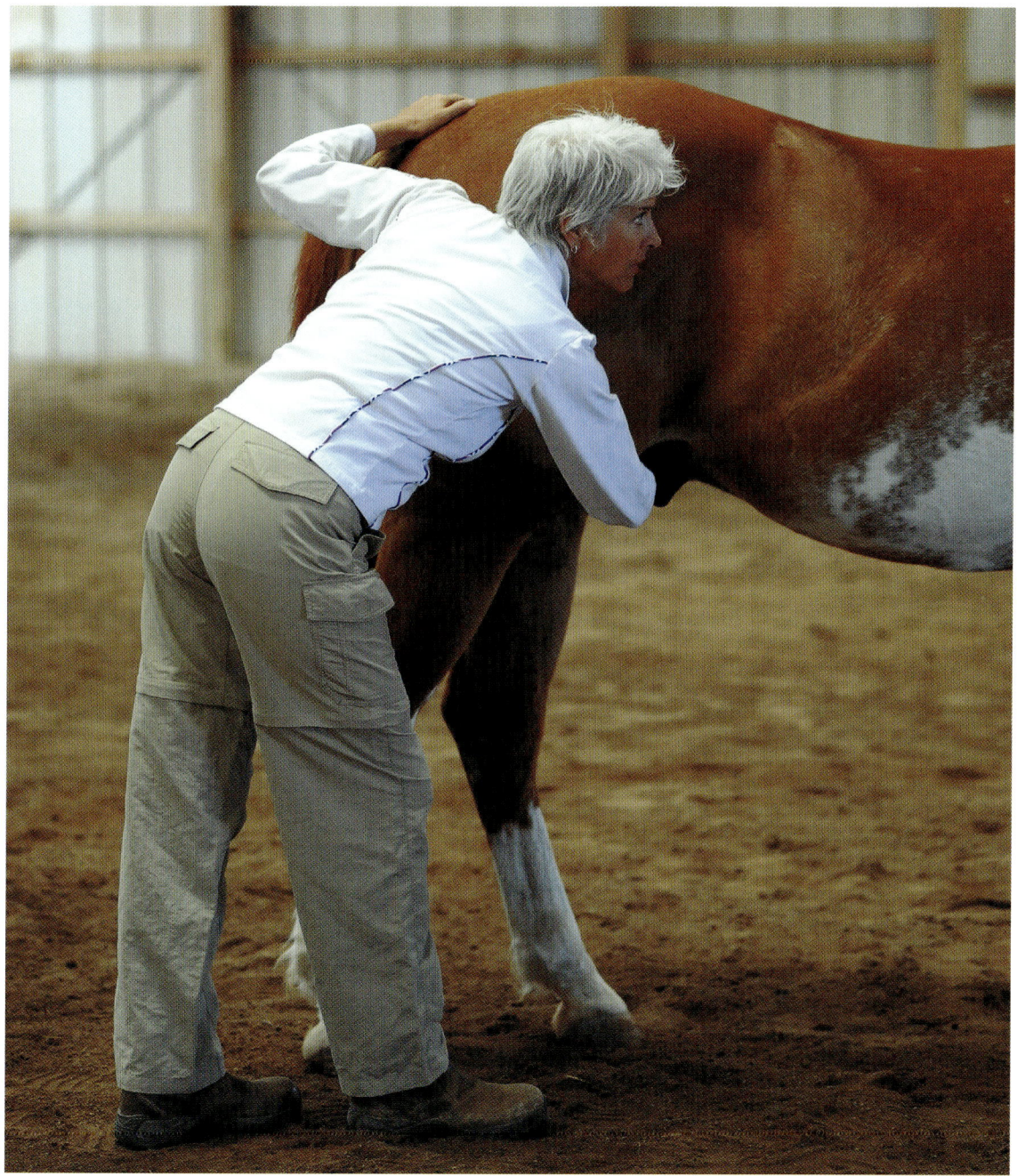

◄ **6.9** I offer CT a gelding scar release. When the testicle tissue is cold, or cooler than the surrounding tissue, there is tight fascia preventing the tissue from having a normal temperature. Hold the tissue gently and wait for the changes, then offer a few more times. It may require a few releases for a full change.

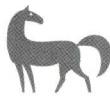

Mystic: The Former Pack Horse

Mystic, an Appendix Quarter Horse mare adopted from a local shelter, was a former pack horse. Her loads had not been evenly balanced. She had strains in her left shoulder, which meant she never took the left lead and wanted to buck instead of canter. Her new owner knew it wasn't a work-ethic problem. We worked on the wooden left shoulder for five sessions, until it melted. The crease finally opened. Her tight withers rose and her sore pectorals opened, letting her feet point straight.

In six more sessions over four months, we released Mystic's sacral and loin areas, as well as her very stiff, clamped tail. Poll and mouth releases transformed her coarse-looking muzzle to a sensitive, delicate profile. Riding focused on the walk and halt, allowing her to balance a human rider instead of a pack load. By the time Mystic had experienced nine months of changes, the saddle maker came to fit a new saddle and complimented Mystic's owner on such a quality Appendix mare. The owner was delighted!

Spreading Conformation Balancing sessions out over at least a six-month time period can allow the horse to balance completely, especially when the rider allows the horse to integrate all the change at the walk before expecting more under saddle.

Canter leads transform. Tight, gelding scar tissue can also completely restrict the horse's hindquarters so that his back must tighten for comfort in his work, which then creates intense sacral/loin strain. I always check the gelding scar for fascial compression.

Neck Imbalance

A concave or "ewe" neck is usually seen as a genetic conformation flaw. Most ewe-type necks result from tight shoulders and withers compression. The solution is to open the entire shoulder, with special care to slowly completely open both the shoulder creases, clear down to the chest.

You then melt the hard fascia along the crest of the neck with a flat palm until the horse is ready for a gentle twisting motion on his neck crest. The tightness inhibits the mane growth, leaving the horse with a sparse or ragged mane.

As you continue to open the neck fascia, pay special attention to the withers, a great tension area. You balance the fascia in the withers, as well, which often requires repeated sessions. It brings great results in topline conformation changes by encouraging an uphill or balanced topline.

Shoulder releases should be repeated regularly to maintain the space (fig. 6.10). As the withers open and rise, the creases stay open as well.

Use strokes in the middle of the neck and open the creases fully, which helps the withers to release, too. At first, the horse's shoulders look somewhat bony and it appears that the horse isn't muscled enough; the new space allows the shoulders to build and the results come as the muscle builds and the shoulders lift. The

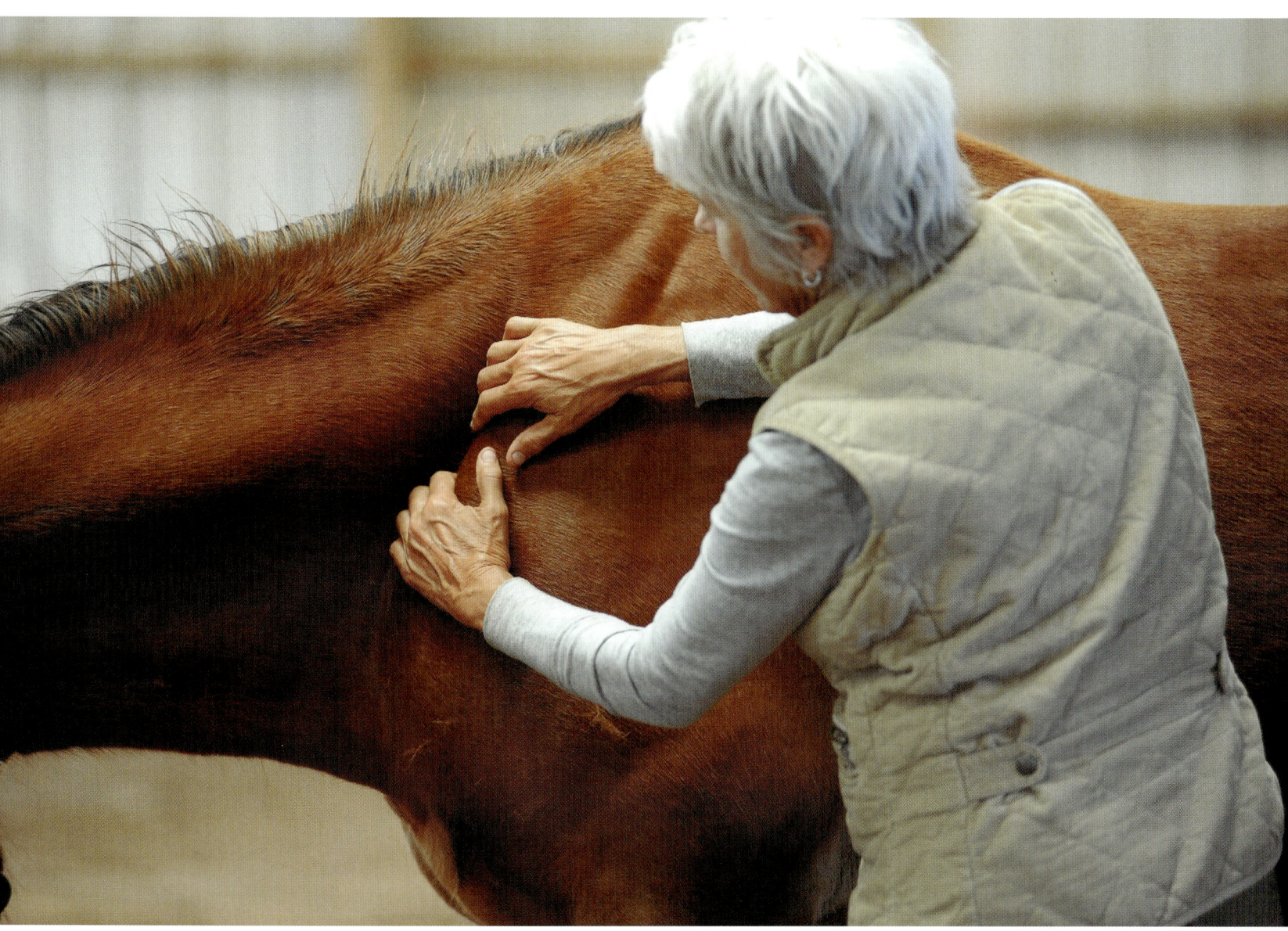

▲ **6.10** This photo shows how to start the shoulder crease opening using the fingers. EZ is lowering his head cooperatively as I slide my fingers into the crease. Gradually, I go deeper and eventually can slip my hand inside.

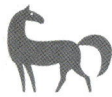

neck curves into a crest, after first becoming level. This change can happen in six months, or even less.

The Gaited Horse

Gaited horses have their own special way of moving. Bred for uneven terrain, the gaited horse served country professionals who traveled long distances daily for customer visits.

Gaited horses benefit from more space and activity and are less likely to develop problems with consistent exercise. The sacral area tends to stiffen without activity; sacral/loin stiffness makes gaiting difficult.

Coffee: He Couldn't Gait

A Rocky Mountain gaited horse, Coffee had lost his gaiting. His hindquarters were tight, and he was cranky. We started in with head releases. While having the front lip release, Coffee circled rapidly for nearly 10 minutes around the corral where we were working. Many circles later, he stopped and enjoyed a very long Still Point before flicking his head to end the release. We finished the session with attention to his tight shoulder creases and tight loins, and did tail releases. After just one session, he found his gaiting and his good humor returned.

An in-mouth release, using all three approaches (see p. 86), helps balance him. The stiff, stuck sacral/loin area makes the horse feel very disorganized, both for himself and the rider.

It's sometimes said these horses have up to 50 or more gaits, and the trick is to get them to do the one the rider wants! In order to find the gaits, the horse has to move on the straight path, without lateral confusion. Then the gaits are more easily identified by both horse and rider. As the horse moves along under saddle, the rider pays close attention, without too much correction, and sorts out what the horse can do. Eventually, with enough riding, the rider can find the most useful and pleasant gaits in the horse.

Riders often forget that the horse usually needs a half-hour of movement to organize. The first 20 to 30 minutes under saddle is best spent by letting the horse move without requesting complicated bends and transitions. As a jogger starts out with a warm-up, so it's true for the horse.

The attentive rider can find what gait speed works best. Gaited horses also do flying lead changes, an additional asset, if the rider can identify it as such. These horses are highly athletic, and often the rider accesses only a small fraction of their talent.

The shoulder creases of a gaited horse must be open and balanced or they have lateral imbalance, which affects gaiting. Both creases should open the same amount. Attention to the sacral and lumbar area of the back helps, as well as keeping the shoulder creases fully opened for front-end freedom. Also, you should always check the tail. A stiff tail limits sacral/lumbar freedom. The gaited horse benefits from regular tail releases and tail pulls.

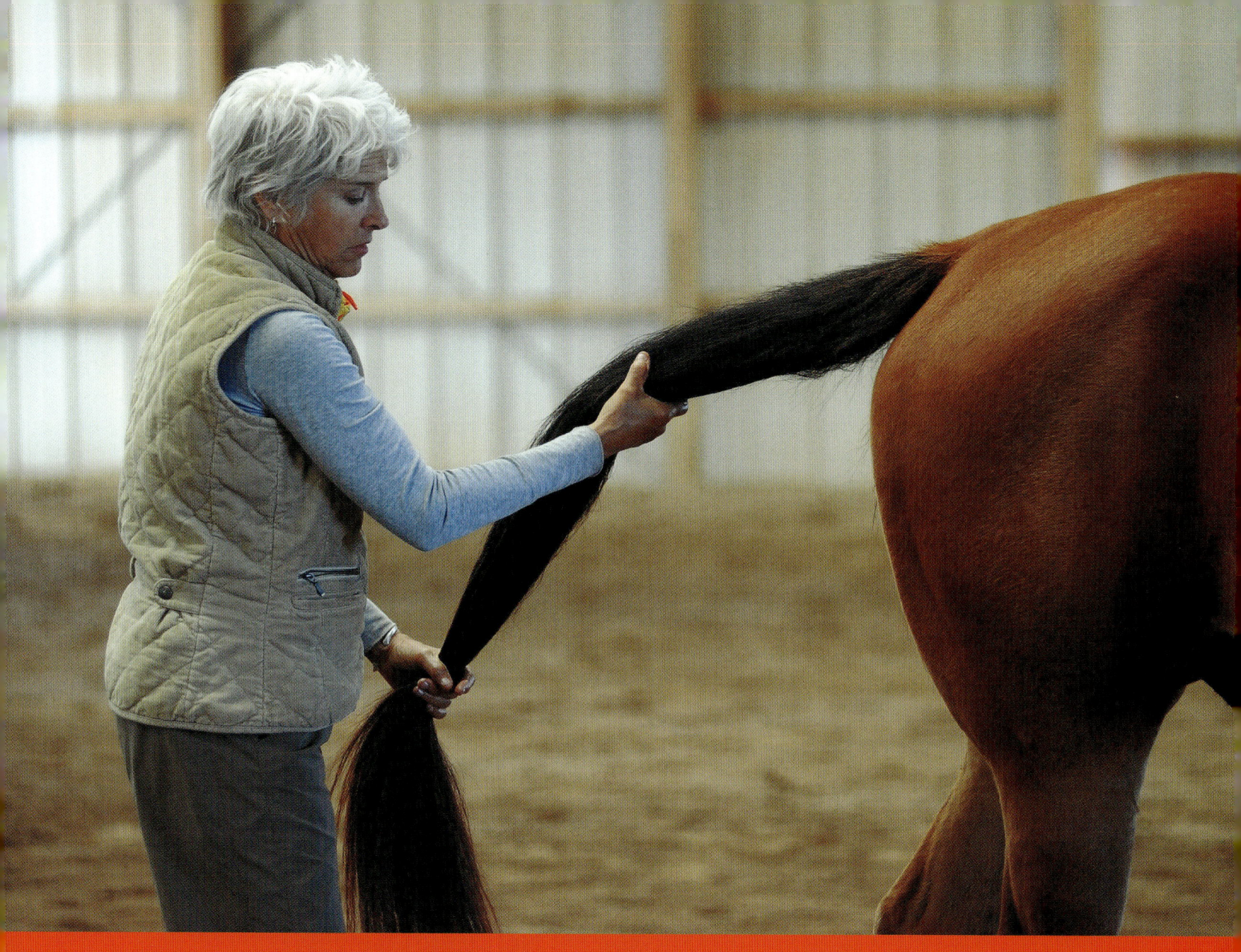

7 | 100% Ability

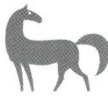

100% Is Possible

The vision of being "100-percent whole" shifted my entire perspective when my body was miserable and stuck. This 100-percent-wholeness vision doesn't mean we know the details of how it happens. It means we allow for the reality that it's *possible*. An important detail here is also that 100-percent wholeness is felt not as a "possibility," it is felt as a "reality."

This might be seen as not "accepting reality" by some. However, "miracles" come to those who want them. Horses, more than humans, move forward without debate when they feel improvements happening to them. If you approach your horse's limits with an open mind, he feels this permission to improve no matter how difficult the problem may be.

Since horses are so brilliantly constructed to hide physical limits, the source of their problem is often elusive. Even in cases where we know what happened, we still do not know how the horse's body compensated or resolved the strain to keep moving.

Tests show the problem, not the body's fascial resolution. It's only much later, when adhesions prevent movement, that the old injuries become obvious problems. The secret of success is that the 100-percent vision finds its solutions. I have been part of horse-and-rider teams who experienced serious injuries that seemed impossible to resolve. Yet, the rider and horse found their way to health and balance again.

A "miracle" means an unplanned, unpredictable success. When I work with horses, this openness to full recovery is always part of my approach. It's helpful not to run diagnostics in your mind, but to stay focused on the actual body.

The first step is to accept the injury or imbalance as much as possible emotionally. Injury reminds you that the body's pain has a purpose. Something needs help. It's not a failure of the body; pain is a request for attention. This insight advances you past feeling trapped in limitation and injury, as if your body is a broken machine.

Once you recognize something needs to be done to help your horse, you search for help. As you use different approaches for the fitness problem, the path is often uneven and unsure. There are many modalities to choose from. I recommend keeping records with dates so you can remember what you did and when. Then, good results are easier to track.

Discouragement comes at times. In fact, discouragement can last for weeks or months while you digest your horse's situation. But, when you finally realize how stiff your horse is and how much he must change to do the work you want, that is the beginning of your new path into fitness.

> The horse shows which areas of fascia-change work interest him most. As we follow these interest areas, the dots connect to restore his "internet" connections.

Notice the Changes

Notice the changes, I was told repeatedly as Steve worked on my chronic imbalances. This became my mantra. This approach also serves well for very elusive fitness problems in horses, where all other modalities have failed. Changes can be small, yet they show you that the horse is, indeed, walking again. Or, maybe the foot is now pointed forward, instead of twisting out when he walks. The tail might be looser. His eye is soft. Tacking-up is easier, since he's starting to feel better. These are all small changes that lead you forward through the recovery period.

Horse people are very devoted to their horses. It's gratifying to see how many owners refuse to give up; like the parents of children, they decide that they will search for answers to their horses' problems. I have seen many owners work long hours online gathering information to help resolve a toxicity problem or put together a team to restore their horses' soundness after a diagnosis of navicular disease.

Each horse that has experienced an unfortunate event or trauma needs his own unique recovery process. The successful horse, without problems, also needs his own unique process of athletic maintenance, not continual repetition of movements, which endlessly limit him.

As you notice the gains, you can relax and leave behind a "limited or unfit" feeling about your horse. Small advances organize into major progress. If the horse can't canter at all, a steady, comfortable trot is an advance. Regular digital conformation photos reinforce good news.

As the horse progresses when returning from chronic injury, don't force his movement or exercise into

your training requirements, or ask him to maintain a former task level promptly. You walk the horse to completely engage and balance his entire body. When the horse spontaneously offers faster gaits or more difficult movements, his readiness to advance is demonstrated.

Grooming: A Fresh Approach

Grooming is a perfect time to do a body scan (see p. 51) to keep track of how your horse feels. Take advantage of this necessary practice to advance your kinesthetic contact. Learn to check over the less usual areas and look for tightness or a "discomfort cue" from the horse (figs. 7.1–7.4). Your new awareness of the internet of fascia gives you a vast complex of interconnected sites to access, and even casual daily contact with your horse's body can be meaningful.

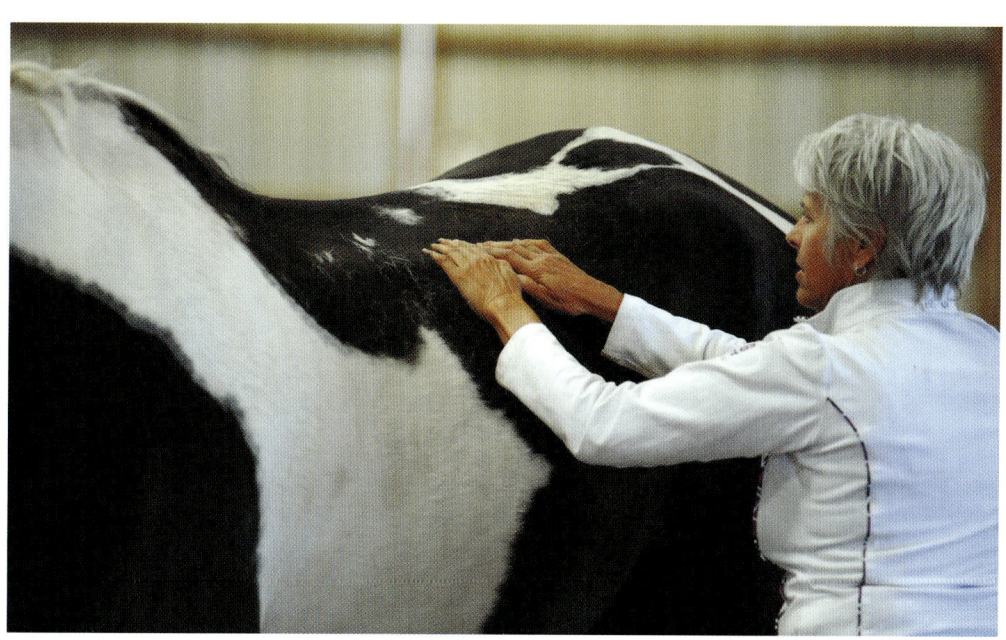

▶ **7.1** My hands sink into Beau's back fascia. This area deserves regular checks on most riding horses to be sure the back is not tightening due to strain.

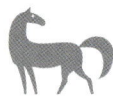

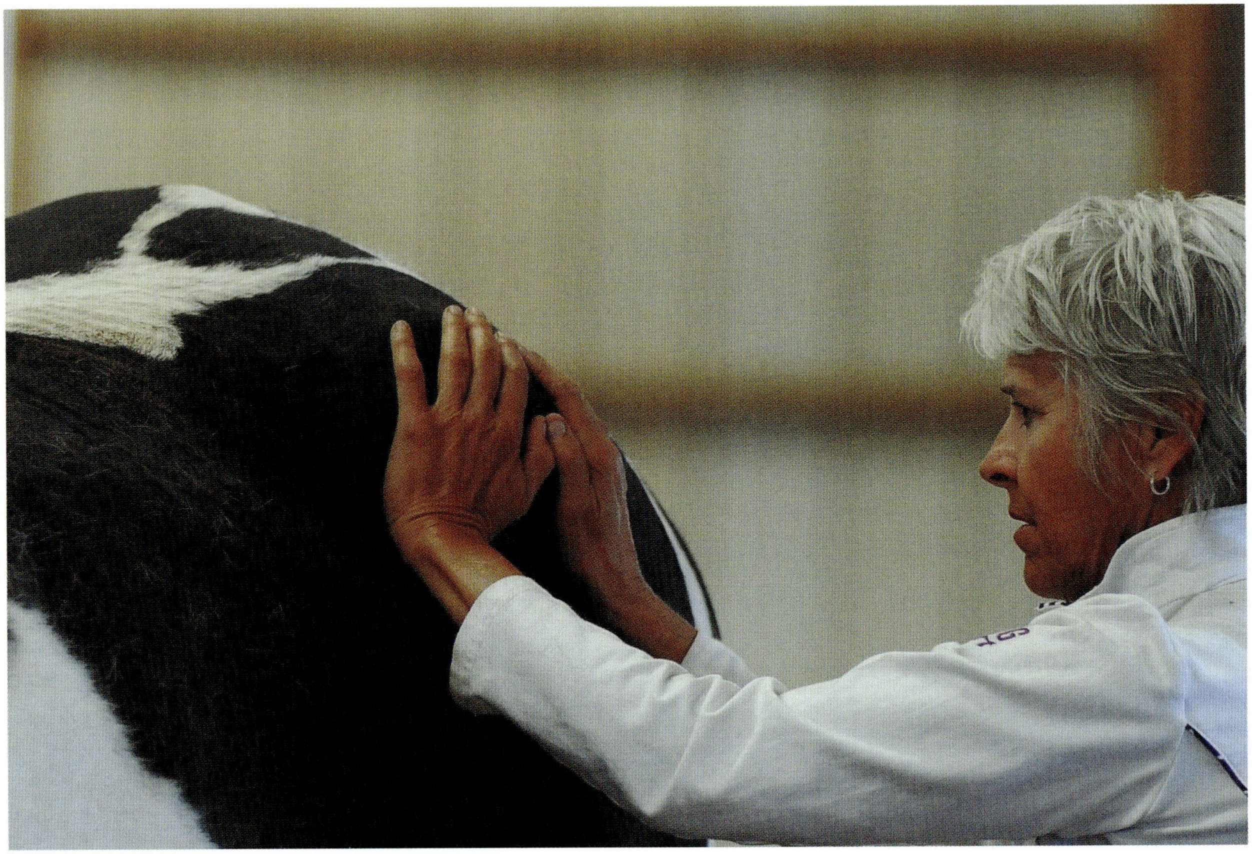

▶ **7.2** Here, I work Beau's compensated hip point, which allows his pelvis to release. This is a routine check-in area for the horse.

Pre-Ride/Post-Ride Check-Ins

- Groom the horse attentively.
- Check the poll; get to know your horse's head.
- Check elbow tightness.
- Shoulder creases.
- Tail tightness and flex; the tail pull.
- Back/loin/sacral check with the palms, before saddling.

In the Saddle

Now that you've noticed the changes and stayed on the recovery path with the horse, what is the best approach for riding work? Turnout is always a good thing, yet it's not a cure-all for lack of movement.

As I noted at the beginning of this book, horses evolved by traveling 50 or more miles per day, over varying terrain. Their natural state of being is *in motion*.

Walk

Recovery and development exercise focuses around the walk. The walk has many speeds and, as noted by horse people worldwide, is the master gait.

Many horses recovering from lost capacity are best conditioned by months of walking at different speeds and over varied terrain. This walk conditioning pays off with big gains in balance and security. Another benefit from extensive riding at the walk is that when the horse's full power returns, both partners are confident in their teamwork, and don't relapse into destructive riding habits, like excessive rein-pulling.

Halt

After the walk, the halt is your second most important tool in the horse's fitness. Your horse's abilities advance as each full-range movement is integrated. The halt, when requested by the rider's seat, restores and develops sacral flexibility and strength. The halt balances the horse gently and effectively, bringing the horse off the forehand, which is an unpleasant result from imbalances and fear.

The halt sensitizes the horse to stopping when your seat shifts, which builds sacral/pelvic/loin strength and the ability to collect. This is progress. A large percentage of horses today are almost frozen in their sacral/lumbar areas (which equate to the human's lower back).

As you know, many riders have lower-back stiffness. The modern sedentary lifestyle is not what we were developed to do, just as the stall or small paddock is not what the horse was evolved to live in. So, we share similar problems: lack of easy, steady movement to keep the back flexible.

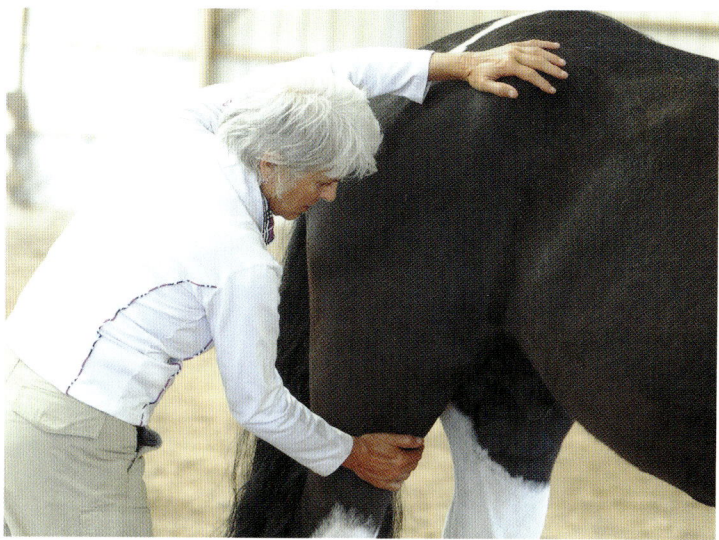

▲ **7.3** The stifle and hip are regular maintenance areas for many horses like Beau, who experience front- and hind-end strain.

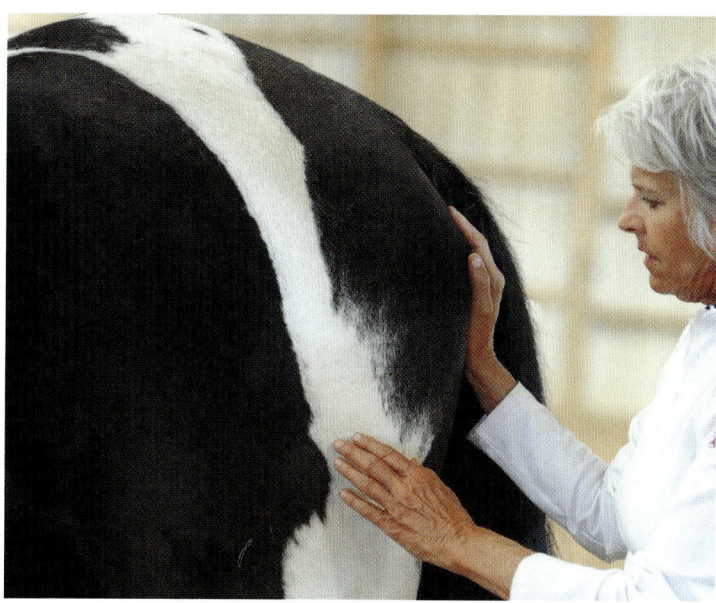

▲ **7.4** The ilium is another area for regular maintenance follow-ups. This can be done before or after rides.

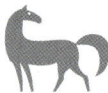

The result is the horse loses the ability to flex in the loin, and pelvic freedom disappears over time. Pelvic freedom is a requirement of collection, along with most other advanced disciplines. As you practice riding at the walk and learning to shift your seat for halts, the horse reconnects with his sacral area. As he identifies the sensations again, he hears your aids and responds. This brings freedom for collection. Many horses are so stiff that true collection is in another universe for them. They don't feel enough to find the muscles to perform it.

Shoulder-In

Another aid to developing sacral strength and balance is the shoulder-in. When it's done correctly, this movement advances the horse's entire hindquarters by building fascial freedom of movement in the sacral juncture, loin, and pelvis. The shoulders and withers also rise easily and naturally in this exercise, when the neck is not allowed to bend, bringing excellent advances to the topline.

Shoulder-in works well for horses of all ages. It is practiced at the walk and the neck should not bend. The crossing of the hind legs develops a "hind consciousness" for the horse, as well as lateral flexion. Many riding books and training approaches teach the shoulder-in. Every rider is encouraged to learn this important movement exercise for maximizing her horse's abilities. It's an easy exercise for practicing a few times weekly while walking. The results will please both you and your horse.

How to Know When to Slow Down

Assess how the horse moves. There are clues to imbalance that show you that movements requiring high training are beyond the horse's present ability. If you are "in training," you need to account for the horse's present ability and not impose a list of training goals on the horse. Like building a house, you don't put wallpaper, paint, or curtains up before the walls are plastered and the wiring is installed.

Signs of Imbalance in the Horse

- Tripping or falling.
- Stopping often during a ride.
- Lowering the head often to balance himself.

Shenny: From Defensive and Dangerous to Pleasant and Safe

Shenny was shot with birdshot, although no one knew how it happened. The small pellets continually worked out of the skin on his neck and head. A talented golden bay Saddlebred, he moved very well. But he was filled with anxiety.

Shenny was very tense at first, but as he realized how Conformation Balancing sessions helped him, he showed full acceptance. In successful monthly sessions over a year's time, Shenny progressed from extreme and dangerous defensiveness to being a pleasant, safe horse for riding and handling.

- Stretching his neck in either direction.

- A twist in the body that prevents straightness.

- Moving on the forehand.

- Inability to stop promptly.

- A twist in his tail, any direction.

Balancing Exercises

- Walk: Start with a moderate walk and progress to varied speeds.

- Halt often on rides, using the seat, not the reins.

- Do hill work, up and down.

- Allow the gallop to precede the canter, if needed, when returning to balance.

- Ride with a loose rein; do not attempt collection until balance comes.

- Shoulder-ins, correctly performed, aid in sacral and pelvic integration.

- Choose tasks that broaden the horse mentally as he regains his abilities.

The Multiplier Effect

If the horse has spent years unfit, it may take up to a year for him to completely balance again, especially if he is talented and has experienced gaps in his training. This is not a "lost year." The horse can now reorganize and gain confidence. It's also a time to learn basics that were missed: tempo, halts, and lightness for both the horse and rider.

Full competency brings a multiplier effect to his capacity, including transforming his attitude into true faith in the rider's judgment, as well as self-confidence and high mental poise. When the horse succeeds in his tasks, he is happier. When he can move well and without pain, this is success. With success at small but basic tasks, he gains confidence in himself—and you as well. You are no longer requesting difficult or impossible movements, you are building out from one athletic strength to add another. Your continual attention to the horse's fascia through Conformation Balancing brings continual physical advance for him.

The Horse's View

Confidence and mental poise in horses are prized qualities. As you facilitate fascial transformation, especially with head and poll changes, the horse finds mental balance. He lives in the present. This is especially important with horses that have been moved many times or had unhappy situations. It is thought by many that these horses come with a form of Post-Traumatic Stress Disorder (PTSD). We all experience the burden of the unhappy past, especially the horse. Without fascial changes, it can take years for a horse to outgrow a miserable life experience, if indeed he ever does leave it behind. With poll and body changes, the horse's mind grows into balance and receptivity each time you offer the contact (figs. 7.5–7.10). Regular sessions transform horses with panic attacks and fearful attitudes.

The more you offer balancing change, the more comfortable your horse's life becomes. Soon, horse-and-rider chemistry blossoms into an enhanced partnership as the horse experiences your compassion and

GROWING INTO BALANCE AND RECEPTIVITY

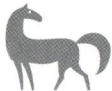

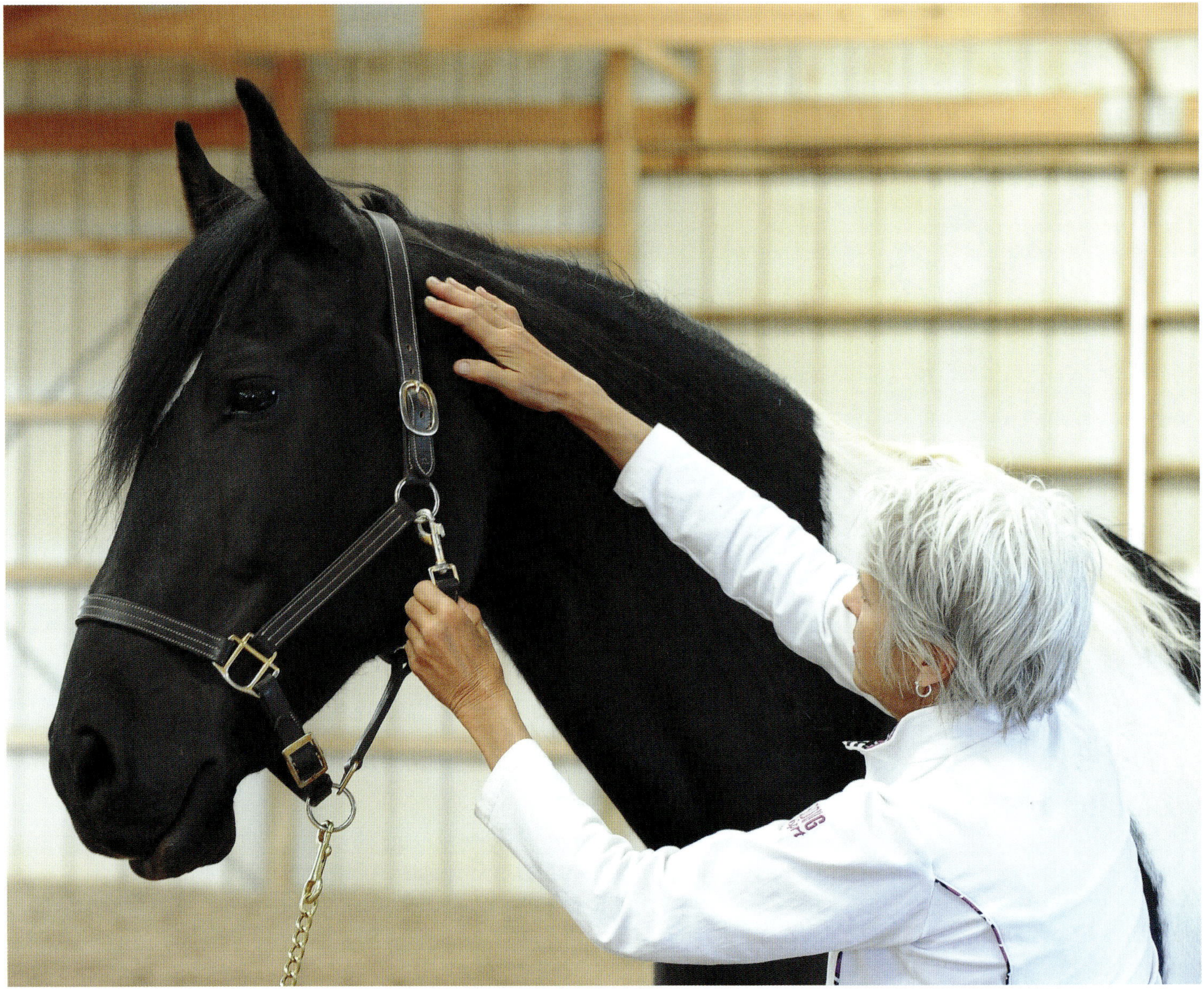

▲ **7.5** Beau has a Still Point with a poll change. A light touch creates huge change, thanks to the interconnectivity of fascia.

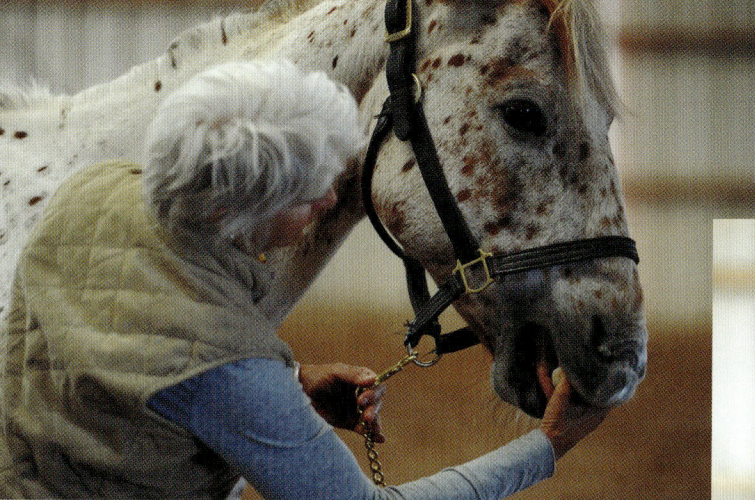

◄ **7.6** Remy has a Still Point with this front lip change. This fascia is often tight and a good maintenance area.

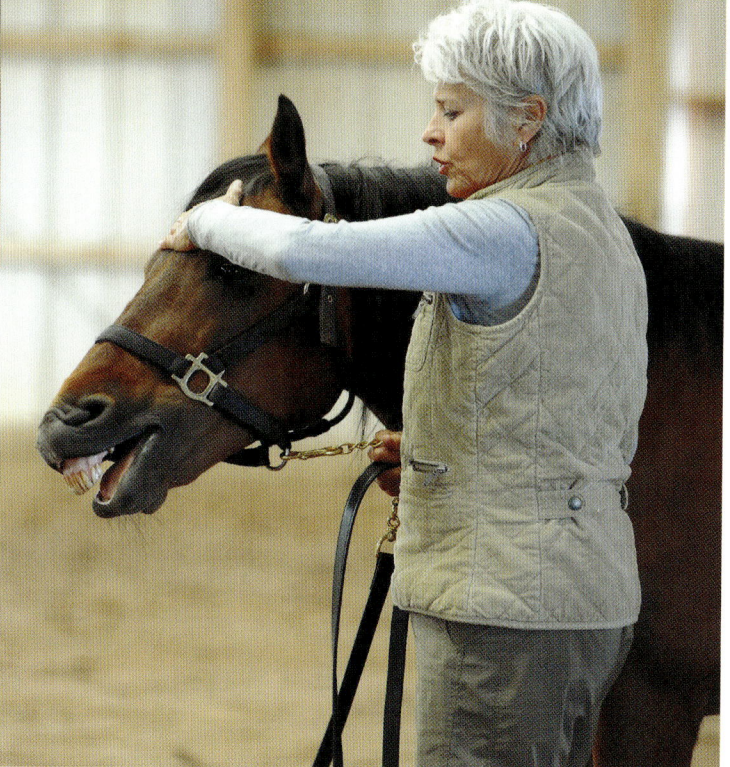

▲ **7.7** Samson shows major response to this forehead release. This balancing is lasting and progressive.

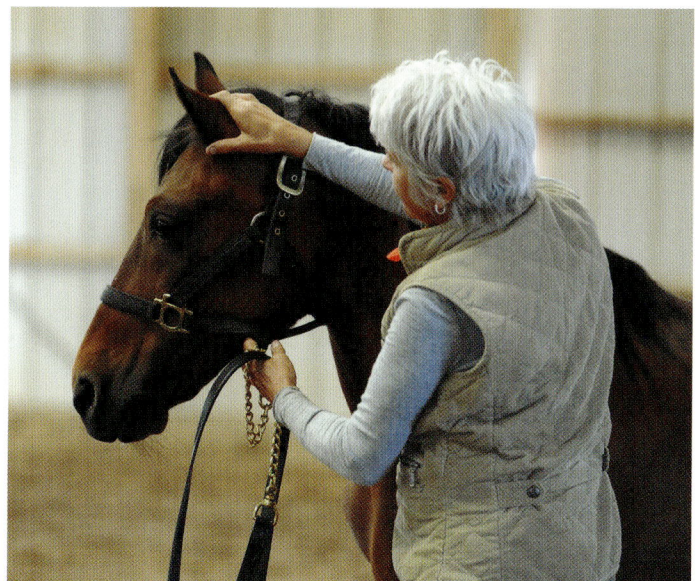

▲ **7. 8** Here, Samson shows a deep Still Point with an ear balancing change. Ears are always on your check-in contact list.

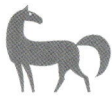

GROWING INTO BALANCE AND RECEPTIVITY (CONTINUED)

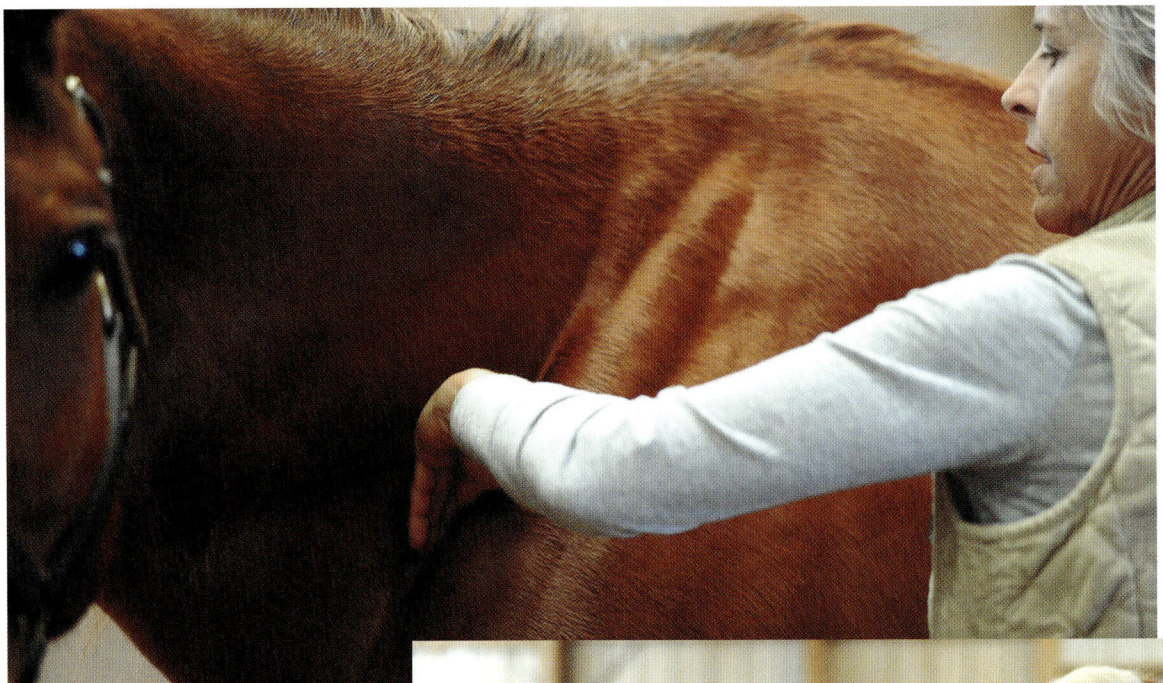

▲ **7.9** EZ's expression shows the connection and trust I am striving for as he enjoys this shoulder crease fascia change.

▶ **7.10** Scout is deep in a Still Point as he receives a poll balancing change. It looks so simple but it brings profoundly effective, lasting results.

willingness to help him with longstanding pain, physical blocks, and fear. You always balance the horse's perspective with your own goals.

If a new stiffness surfaces, continue to balance stuck areas of fascia for free movement. The limits surfacing were present but hidden, costing the horse energy and athletic ability. A major question occasionally surfaces as well: are you ambivalent about the horse's fitness? Only the rider can answer this question.

Conformation Balancing might seem frustrating in relation to your riding goals until you truly realize that the problems *are there*; you will face them again and again, especially in challenging situations, until they are resolved. The good news is that with each Conformation Balancing advance, stability comes and progresses ever further with more permanence.

With any fascia-fitness progress, the horse enjoys the "multiplier effect." He feels a lot better with just a few contact sessions. Topline transformations come very quickly now. This visual progress assures you, even besides the improvement in your rides, that the horse is truly becoming more himself and advancing his skills.

"One-and-Done" Fails

The nature of fascia, as I've discussed throughout this book, shows you why one fix doesn't return the horse to full fitness. Fitness for the horse—like the rider—is ongoing. If the rider has a "one-and-done" approach to fitness, she will never enjoy the peace of progress with her horse. The one-and-done approach leaves both horse and rider at a substandard performance level with deteriorating abilities.

Just as you don't keep your fitness without continual vigilance, neither does the horse. The major difference is that the horse is often well over 900 pounds; accidents are devastating to all concerned. The point for ongoing balancing of fascia is to advance athletic competency, despite circumstances. With competency, the horse stays sound and fit easily for many years of productive, enjoyable riding.

> When a relapse occurs, just say, "Okay! There's more balancing to do!"

Each relapse is actually an opportunity to find true fitness. The dreaded result of unsoundness is a damaged horse, now doomed to pasture or, worse, forced into extended inactivity in the boarding barn environment. An important factor to consider is that "downtime," when the horse is not fit or able to be active in your sport, requires resources. It's an efficiency to keep the horse moving well and happily.

Relapses occur when hidden tightness and compensations remain. Relapse also occurs when you ask for too much too soon in the recovery process. Slow progress is more effective than presuming the horse is well because he looks better. In cases of chronic imbalance, the horse often needs to learn to move competently again and find all his abilities. Often, after a long period of sustained injury—which might be three to five years or more—the horse has become quite numb, and has lost his sense of easy movement. He doesn't move well yet, and like the recovering jogger, doesn't choose the hardest hills right away. Impatience for results is an enemy of progress.

Riders that purchase horses from shelters and

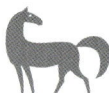

situations of extended idleness often find that the horse is not athletic and is unresponsive in major parts of his body. These horses respond very well to Conformation Balancing and the development process presented here.

The key is to not hurry or insist on specific, technical tasks early. The best approach is to simply ride and discover what the horse has, while offering all the methods for fascial change in this book. These "rehab horses" often bring many years of pleasure and service to their new owner, once their old limits are released.

Topaz: The Pony That Loved Polo

The polo pony's elusive injuries were hard to find. More than a few professionals couldn't locate the source of the problem. I offered him long sessions for three days in a row and began to find deep fascial compensations in the left shoulder and right hind.

Topaz loved his sport, and it was hard to hold him back to just a walk about the field and around the game. As he improved with intensive sessions over three months, his owner began to take him to matches—but he got excited and overworked in that environment. After a few days, he became lame again. The answer was to allow him several months off in a 40-acre pasture to walk at his own pace as much as he chose. Topaz returned fully to fitness, his owner carefully regulating his work ethic, within a year.

Full Competency: Is the Rider Ready?

A fully competent horse—100-percent-whole—is extremely athletic. Anyone who's watched jumping, racing, barrel racing, or other equine sports knows how amazingly the horses rebalance from potential disaster. The crowd sighs collectively in relief when a jump is successful despite unfavorable timing or takeoff. We all want success and safety for the horses—and the riders!

Full competency creates athletic successes. Even small limitations result in loss of athletic ability. Adversities such as mud, rider errors, other competitors, varied footing, travel exhaustion, or weather changes require the horse to organize his own competency to negotiate his success. It's easy to forget that any one of these factors can be the tipping point.

What about the rider's conditioning? Another honest assessment here is vital for the rider/horse team. Let's look at some basics regarding the rider.

Rider Checklist

- Are you fit yourself? What are your own stuck, injured areas?

- Are you realistic in your goals for yourself?

- Is your impatience really a way to camouflage fear?

- Do you enjoy resolving problems in your horse and yourself?

- Can you approach rides creatively and respond to the horse's needs?

- Can you discipline advanced goals to an appropriate timeline?

- What are true rider goals?

- Is your current horse really suitable for your needs?

Once you know the horse's body better, you can then match your own goals with your horse's situation. If the horse isn't ready for competition and that's your honest goal, you have a choice: find a new horse or re-evaluate your goal. If your horse is your "significant other," then his abilities and situation guide you in your riding goals.

Your own lifestyle choices are yet another factor in your riding. City barn, country barn, or at-home boarding situations all bring different opportunities and options for horse and rider. Perhaps riding in hills isn't possible because you live in flat country. Or maybe you don't trailer to other locations. All these factors determine your path. Not to worry, it all works out if you keep an open mind to solutions. As the horse grows in poise, balance, and happiness, he attracts opportunities.

After checking on your own fitness, let's look at your equipment. When the horse changes, tack needs reevaluation. Also, your riding may have changed, requiring new tack. Before running out for a new saddle or gear, take a careful look at what you have and notice how much your horse is changing and *how* he is changing.

Basic Changes in the Horse That Affect Tack Fit and Type

- Withers rise and widen; saddles may fit differently.

- Shoulders open; saddles may fit differently.

- Is the saddle too heavy or too long? Weight on the loins creates strain.

- Sweat patterns become normal; is a gel pad helpful?

- The head changes shape; browbands don't fit.

- The poll is softer; is the old bit too severe and heavy?

- Is the saddle responsive to the horse's new back?

- Do you use heavy reins on a soft mouth and an easily flexing neck?

- Is a noseband necessary?

- Revisit shoeing habits; the hooves may have changed.

- Are you choosing different kinds of riding exercises? Do you have new goals?

During the Conformation Balancing process, it's not the right time to fit a custom saddle. Even the highest quality saddle may not fit the horse after conformation changes. When the horse is changing, wait on saddle purchases for at least three months, if possible. It's best to find a saddle that works rather than ordering one that might be outdated in less than a year.

Horses with narrow-looking withers often become much broader once the shoulders/withers juncture is fully released. Horses with fatty mutton withers often shrink to medium width when their shoulders are opened and balanced with muscle development. High withers may disappear as the neck develops and the shoulders open fully. A horse that never sweats much may suddenly come home soaking wet after medium exercise.

The browband should not fit tightly around the ears, but many horses become broad in the brow after cranial change and a stock-sized browband no longer fits well. Split-ear headstalls deserve a careful look. A tight fit around one ear changes the fascia for that ear, as well as the poll.

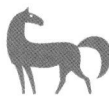

Nosebands also need examination for tightness, as well as a flash that is often buckled tightly around the horse's nose. A tight flash cuts circulation and changes fascial patterns, as well as impacting tongue, jaw, and mouth fascia. Fascia changes in the mouth and nose can, and often do, affect the horse's head balance in long- and short-term ways.

Bits with long shafts put great leverage on the poll and jaw. When the rider is not light-handed, this unbalances the horse continually. The horse loses poll softness if his head is bent down with the bit. True poll softness results from the poll having freedom to bend and the jaw being open enough to flex. True collection always results from hind end impulsion.

Hooves change with Conformation Balancing. Do the shoes still work? Can the horse go barefoot now? Have the feet changed? Often, flares in hooves disappear following balancing. Stiff, heavy feet actually shrink and become normal as the hoof fiber, which is keratin, like hair, becomes flexible as the horse moves better. Horses that stand around miserably due to body stiffness develop hoof problems that often disappear as they regain balance. Many farriers are amazed and pleased at the hoof changes for the horse after six months of Conformation Balancing. A year later, they don't recognize the horse.

If the horse is being returned to competency and integration, training goals are not the priority until he has truly integrated his physical gains. A horse without balance and fitness is not a capable candidate for collection, jumping, or other competitive athletic goals. These activities are for fit horses, not horses growing *toward* fitness. A horse that has experienced complete or partial breakdown through injury or poor development needs time to learn his body's abilities again. "Hurry" short-circuits the horse's achievement of competency, as noted earlier. Unfortunately, sometimes, the blame is put on bodywork or muscle development as being inadequate. You must recognize that hurrying the process to run a race on a healing leg can end everything!

HORSE COMPETENCY CHECKLIST

- The horse is poised and confident.
- Tacking up is easy: no girth or headstall problems.
- The horse stops well, on the flat and hills.
- The horse is not on the forehand.
- There aren't patches of ruffled hair on gaskins, flanks, or shoulders.
- The horse bends his poll easily.
- The horse has stamina and can work easily.
- Sweat patterns are normal and healthy.
- Hooves wear evenly; shoe wear is also even.
- The horse bends evenly on both sides.
- The horse stands square often and easily.

Fitness Is a Process, Not a Goal

Fitness is an ongoing, constantly changing relationship with your body. As a rider, this ongoing personal relationship expands to include a large animal. The human world thrives on using machines, data, and other technological or mechanical tools to accomplish and measure progress. With horses, it's still a partnership process even though we use time, specifications, and other devices to measure success. We tend to rely on repetition for our achievements. This seems to work, until it doesn't. If the horse has strain, even without our knowing it, compensations are happening constantly.

The body is not static. It is either improving or growing less competent. This means that, despite the aging process, the horse is either becoming fit or less fit. Fitness means that the horse meets his life with competency, no matter what circumstances he encounters. We can't create perfectly safe lives for our horses, and indeed, even if we could, that would not be an advantage.

Variation keeps us growing. As you know, arena training does not stimulate the horse's ability to handle rough ground or slopes. Cross-training is always sought in the sports world, including horses.

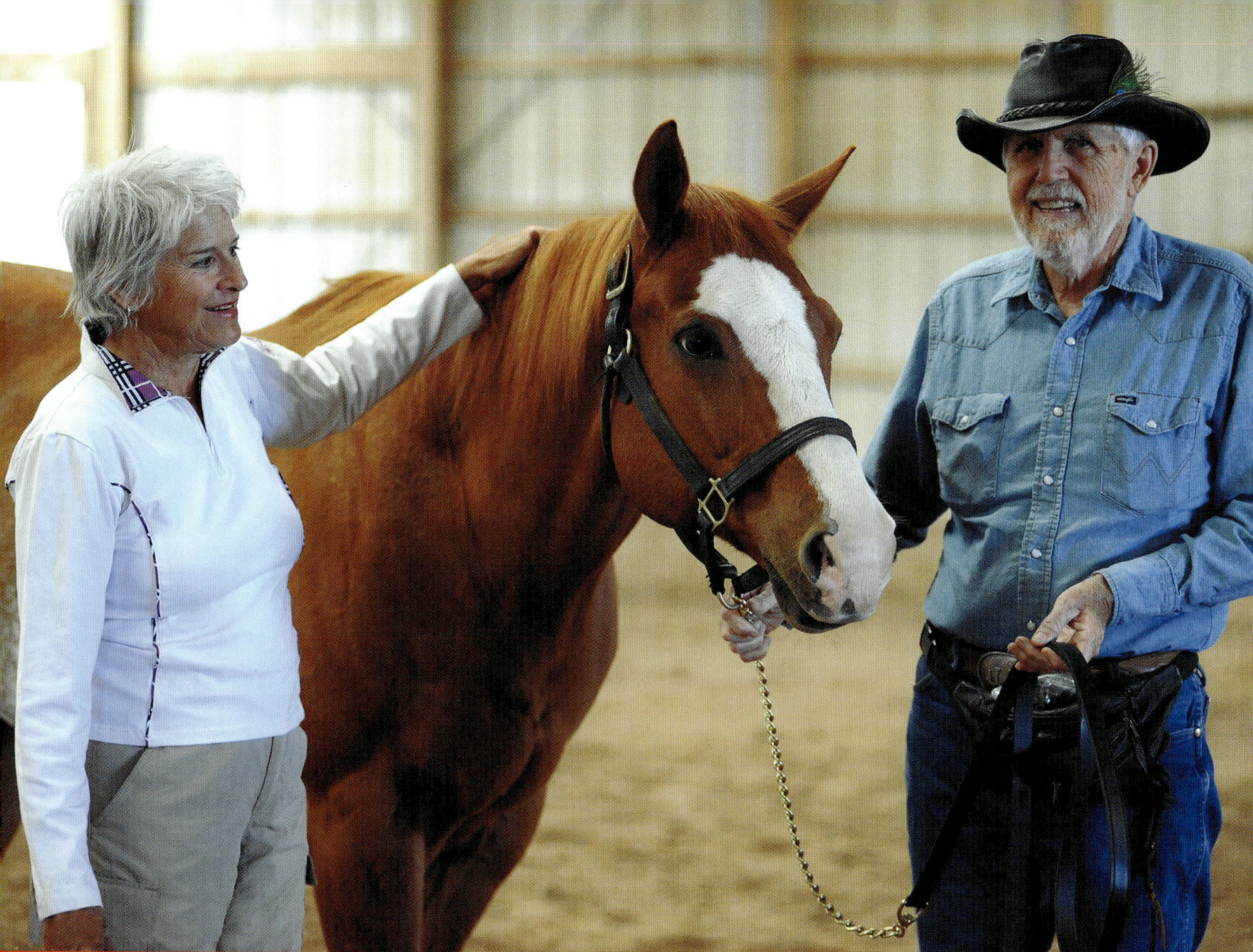

8 | A Happy Horse
Is Priceless

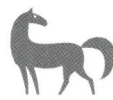

Garre: A Horse with High Standards

Garre was exquisitely bred and had been trained to Grand Prix dressage by age 11. His history also included jumping. When his owner called me to work with him, she said her own therapist had recommended fascia-change work for Garre's issues, which included a long-term stifle problem.

Garre was angry and defensive. It was easy to see why. He was lightly built and he now had difficulty even with basic collection. He was guarding constantly. It took five sessions before I could touch his stifle.

But then Garre became a most willing client. We resolved many compensations from three serious injuries that were the result of a jumping accident and the beginning of his troubles. Poll and head balancing were a turning point for Garre. His temperament improved vastly, and he became a safe and willing riding partner again.

Garre shows how important it is to work at the horse's pace and proceed at the horse's acceptance. His sessions were weekly for eight weeks, with all riding at walk and trot only. Sessions decreased to twice monthly for another two months. His owner waited for recovery of the stifle before returning to canter work under saddle. The guarding had improved within a month's time and tacking up became possible without incident. The light work allowed Garre to relax, and he "unwound," releasing mental tension as his head balanced.

Now, a few years later, after about 24 sessions, Garre is once again peforming dressage tests happily with his rider. You follow the cues to find the most efficient and safe path to fitness at the horse's pace.

The Critic Is Not Your Friend

Our inner (or outer) critic likes to tell us the horse is not improving and Conformation Balancing takes too long. Or, maybe the critic says your horse is not built well and doesn't have what it takes. This is seldom true. Nearly all horses today are well built and have plenty of physical ability, unless the rider chooses a highly specialized sport, such as jumping.

Poor quality horses are removed from the gene pool quickly by circumstances and intentional selection. If you remember, about 100 years ago, the horse was mankind's mode of transportation. Any fit, healthy horse was an asset, no matter if he was built well or not. The coming of motor vehicles brought new roles for the horse: recreation and sports. This change removed many of the horses considered unattractive, unless they had special talent, a great personality, or were in distant locations from the market. Today, nearly every horse has reasonably balanced conformation.

How Long?

Back to that old question: How long does it take? It takes what it takes, as I was told myself, when I first started on this path. If you learn to enjoy the changes as they come, you find plenty of motivation for this fitness process. Whether your concerns are recovery, maintenance, or progress, this Conformation Balancing approach to fitness brings security in its rewards. You will truly *know* your horse.

When a glitch comes, you'll feel ready to see it clearly. A recovery process for a horse injury can go many different ways. Frustration occurs when a single approach to full recovery doesn't happen. A combination of supportive approaches to any fitness problem brings the best results.

When you follow the fascial internet patiently, you'll eventually find all the "sites" that are blocked by stiffness or adhesions. You maintain a moderate activity and exercise routine for the horse. Feeding and foot care also are part of the plan. If you desire prompt gains, fascia-change work is best used weekly, or whenever the horse permits it. Moderate gains occur at a monthly session rate. When the sessions are widely spaced, change is slower. The easiest way to progress is consistent weekly or twice weekly contact on any area that shows limits. Many short sessions will advance the horse much more quickly, as well as resolving mental anxiety so that rides are much more pleasurable for horse and rider. Again, a photo record will remind you of the changes (see p. 34).

> Notice the changes: Practice seeing the horse's gains.

"Can't" Not "Won't": The Horse Is Trying

Horses live with constantly changing weather, work conditions, varied tack, hauling, rough social companions, and maybe even different riders. All these factors make consistency of movement a challenge. Their personal lives are usually hidden from your view and accidents happen without you ever knowing about them. The mysterious loss of ability surfaces like an enemy in your rides or training.

The horse needs your support here, not pressure to perform his old tasks easily. He often cannot. You return to the fact that the horse usually *can't* do it rather than *won't* do it. He obviously doesn't watch movies, read books, or look at computers. He stays present with his body all day. When something isn't feeling good, it's a problem. Stuck fascia brings difficult days where the horse dreads his work.

This new information about the internet of fascia lets you look more closely at the horse's conformation and pay attention when you ride. Rather than thinking that his gait is just about his training, look for internal causes for why he is slow, lacks tempo, moves on the forehand, or any other problem you are working to change. Knowing about fascia means that you know that there are millions, if not billions or trillions, of tiny parts not working smoothly.

As you are helping the horse return to balance, and hopefully improving your own riding as well, Soma-Emotional Recall comes often, at first. As the horse revisits his old history, it's important to allow him to digest this new self he's discovering. Each Soma recall of an old event frees space in his receptivity for new poise and new tasks.

Losses Become Gains

The new freedom in movement lights up the relationship. This is the truth of Conformation Balancing. This process raises the consciousness of the horse by opening his mind to positive recognition of his own progressive abilities to change. Suddenly, life becomes comfortable for him and he lives peacefully in his own skin again. And, like any recovery, peace and service bring happiness.

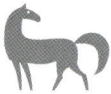

What makes this process so rewarding is that the horse himself is conscious of his change of circumstances. He recognizes his new ability and freedom from pain, and your role in helping him has also qualified you further as a trustworthy leader. The alpha-dominant position is not hard to maintain when you are steadily advancing your horse's health. He knows he can't do this for himself. This new rider role supports your leadership status. The horse is grateful to be on a team where he can relax and be comfortable (figs. 8.1–8.10). What seemed to be a physical loss that would never resolve has now become a relationship asset due to the new trust on both sides.

A fit horse offers more impulsion, more energy, and more power. We know that suitability of work is a vital factor in maintaining athletic competency. Now that the horse's body is waking up and his mind is becoming more conscious, he has much more receptivity to new tasks and problems. This new "intelligence" brings a new level of challenge and possibilities. Horses that showed little academic ability previously often display new patience for high-school work after they progress into a fluid, flexible body.

This is a good time to reassess training methods. Small round pens and other highly structured training methods are not suitable for developing balance in horses. These methods compress fascia tightly with repetitive movement, similar to your own repetitive keyboarding issues.

In the case of young horses, under five years of age, repetitive work nearly always leads to loss of fitness when the horse reaches his mid-teens. As already mentioned, longeing young horses has many side effects: the common practice of longeing a young horse on a single line in a 10-meter circle can cause the horse to fall. This training method deserves a serious look. The transitory gains should be weighed against truly lasting damage to the poll, axis, atlas, and occiput.

Martina: A Complicated Story

Martina, an 11-year-old Quarter Horse/Arabian cross, was purchased for trail riding. All seemed well in the pre-purchase ride, but when the new owner took her out for trail rides, Martina was full of anxiety and often bolted. Her body showed a complicated story. Her short neck lacked any crest. Her poll was very unbalanced and much higher on one side. Her elbows were jammed into her ribs. Her eye had the white ring of fear. In her old safe arena, none of the fear showed, but the new environment, which lacked rows of stables and white fencing, terrified her.

Poll and head balancing produced dramatic changes for Martina. Over three months, 10 Conformation Balancing sessions focused on her head, poll, tight shoulders, and sacral juncture, and she was ridden only at the walk. She had many Still Points and the extreme panic, which her intelligent personality couldn't hide, dissipated over the weeks. She learned to come off her forehand with her rider's patient work at the walk and halt, and Martina transformed into an attractive mare with a soft eye—and she no longer bolted.

BEAU'S CHANGES: A PHOTO JOURNAL

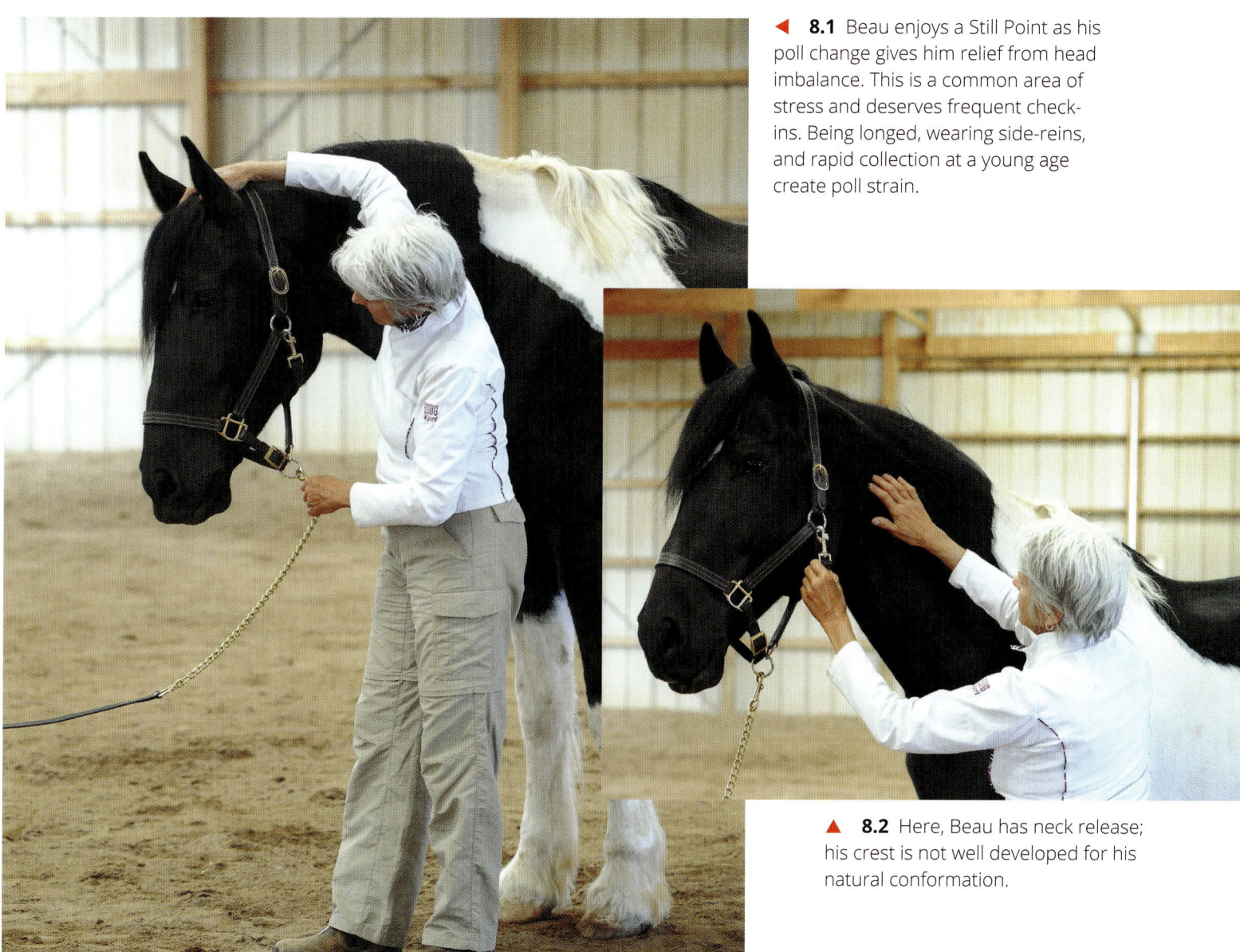

◄ **8.1** Beau enjoys a Still Point as his poll change gives him relief from head imbalance. This is a common area of stress and deserves frequent check-ins. Being longed, wearing side-reins, and rapid collection at a young age create poll strain.

▲ **8.2** Here, Beau has neck release; his crest is not well developed for his natural conformation.

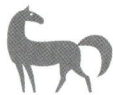

BEAU'S CHANGES: A PHOTO JOURNAL (CONTINUED)

▶ **8.3** Beau sinks into a Still Point with an ear release. Beau's poll strain contributed to his hindquarters unsoundness.

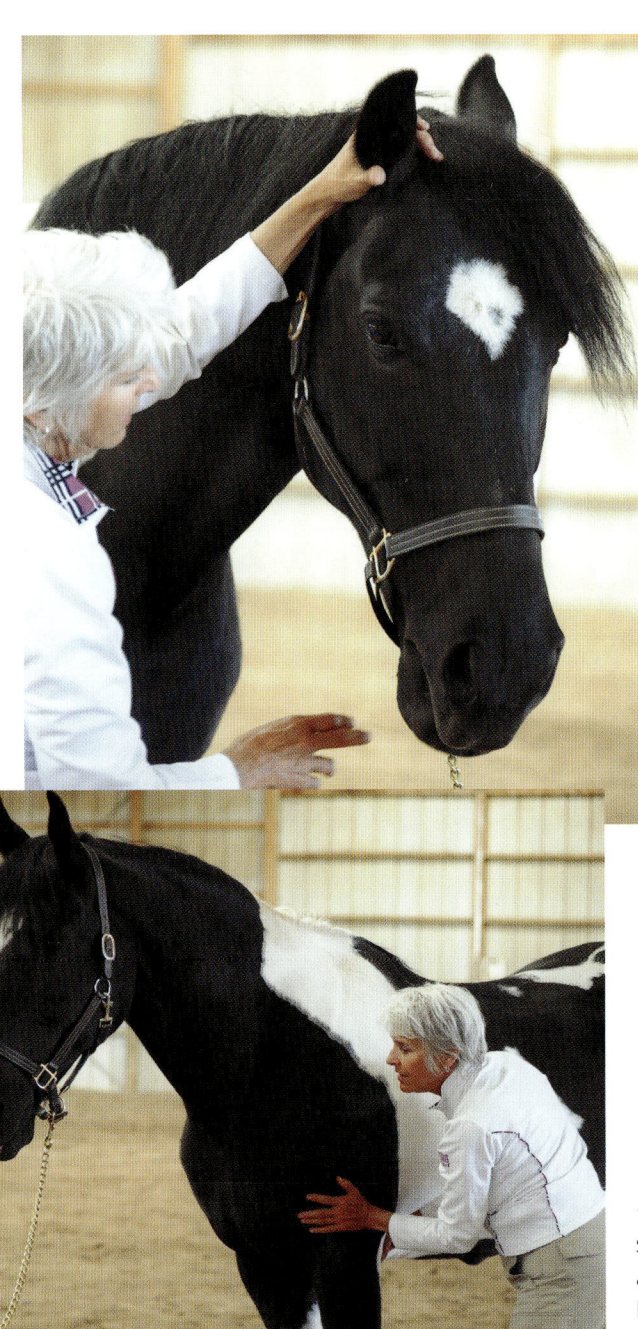

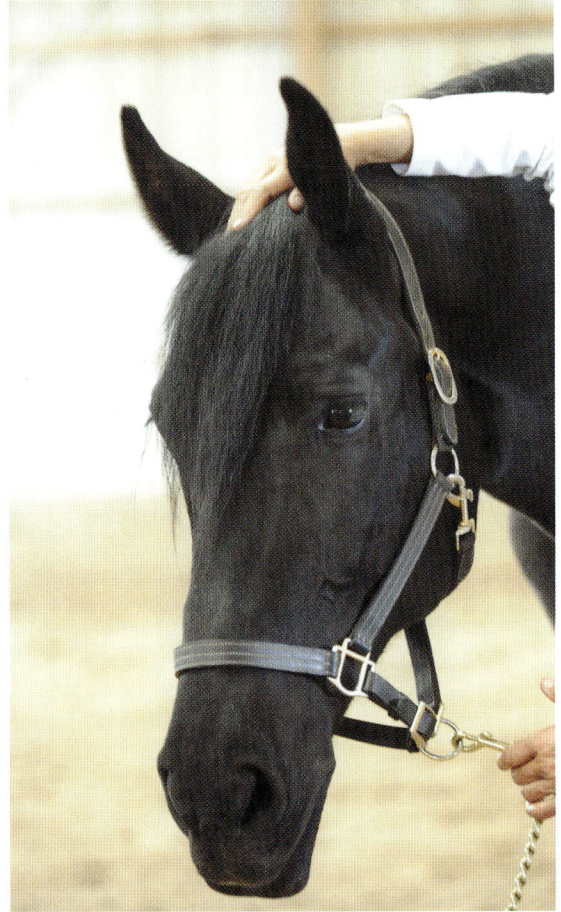

▲ **8.4** Beau enjoys a Still Point with this poll release. The internet of fascia assures me that all "sites" are being reached.

◀ **8.5** The elbow is crucial to ease of stride. The elbow often compensates for a very tight scapula or shoulder and may be so tight that sliding a hand in is very difficult at first. Beau enjoys the change.

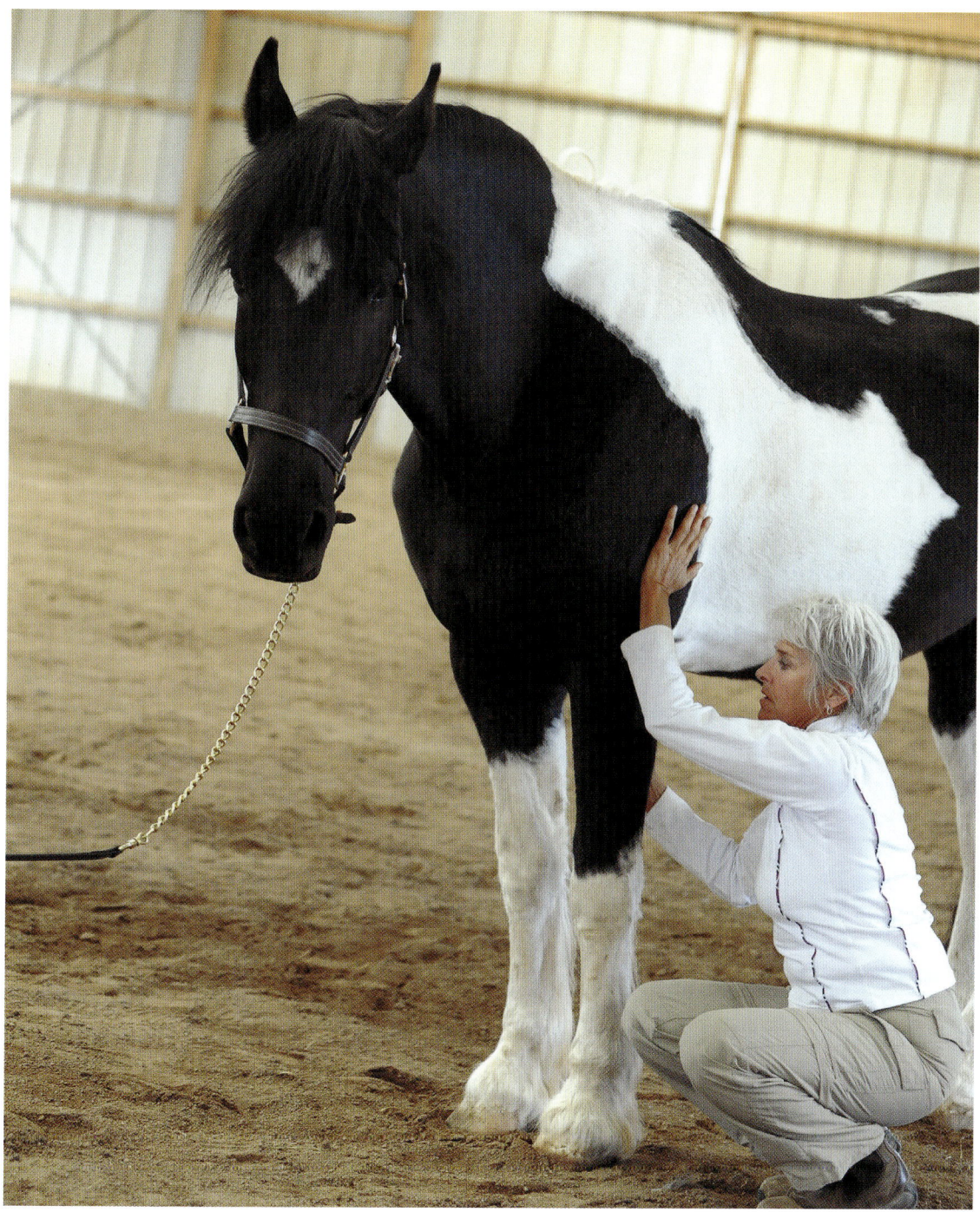

◄ **8.6** Here, I open the shoulder further and also wrap the back of Beau's foreleg. Checking the legs with attentive contact helps find minor compensations. Notice his attention to the change.

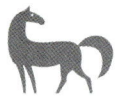

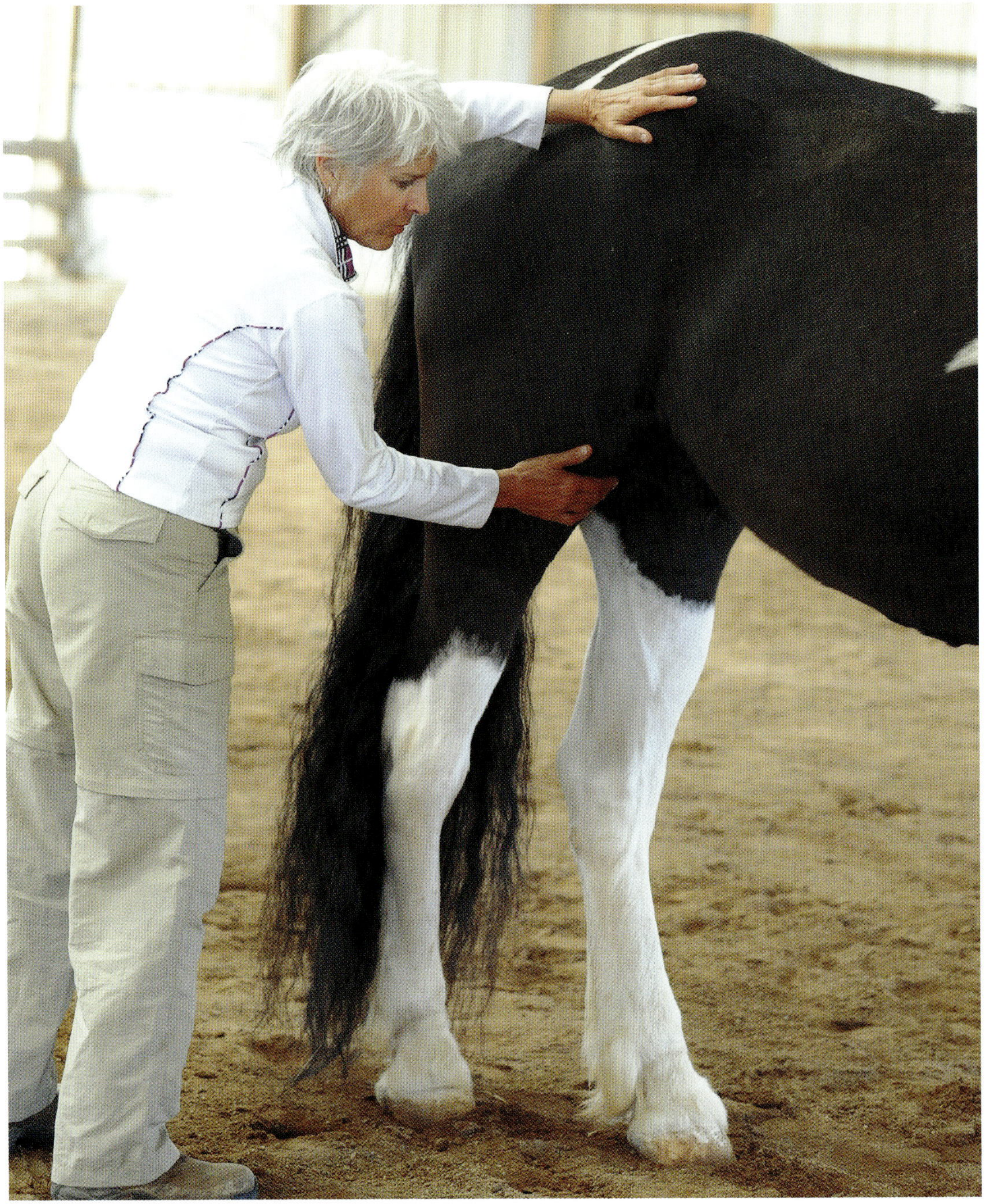

BEAU'S CHANGES: A PHOTO JOURNAL (CONTINUED)

▶ **8.7** Careful, soft palming opens stifle fascia without stress or pain for the horse. I stand at the side, able to step away easily.

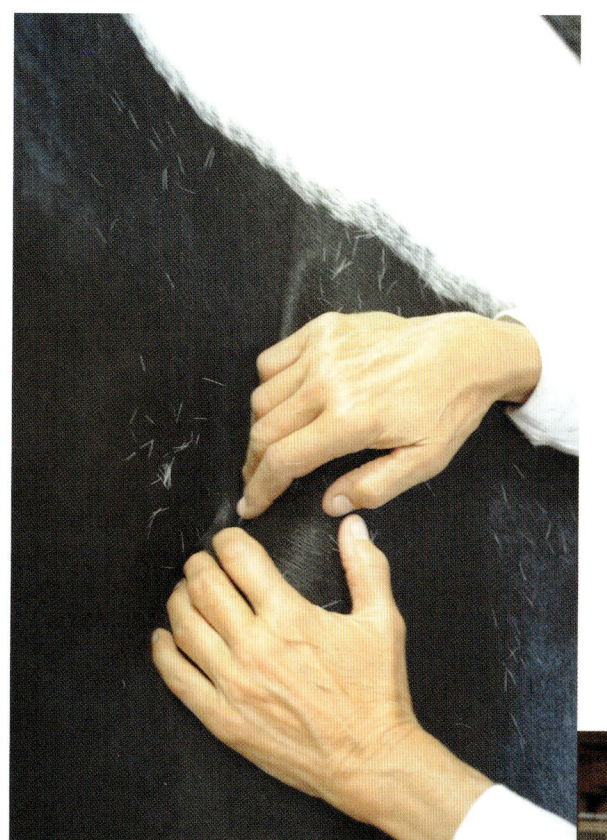

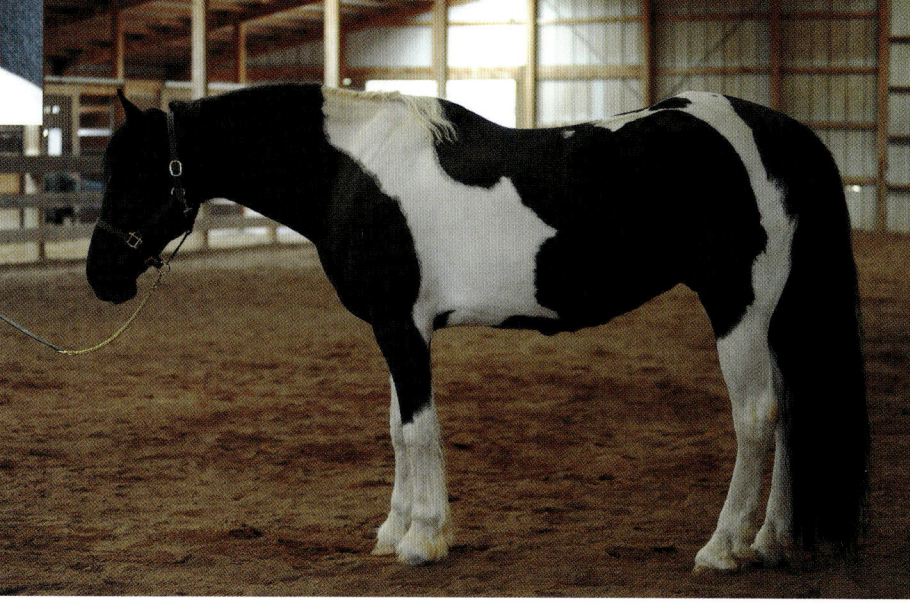

▲ **8.9** Beau is in a Still Point here as I open his shoulder crease. An open shoulder crease is vital to raising the withers and letting the neck crest.

▲ **8.8** The shoulder crease release opens the scapula or shoulder so it moves freely. The shoulder is not attached to the skeleton; the horse has "four-wheel-drive" action on his front end. His shoulder is the center of his gravity. My fingers creep into Beau's tight crease gently.

▶ **8.10** After his session, Beau stands more squarely. His head has dropped and his withers are rising. Digital photos show before and after changes in the horse.

BEAU'S CHANGES: A PHOTO JOURNAL (CONTINUED)

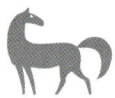

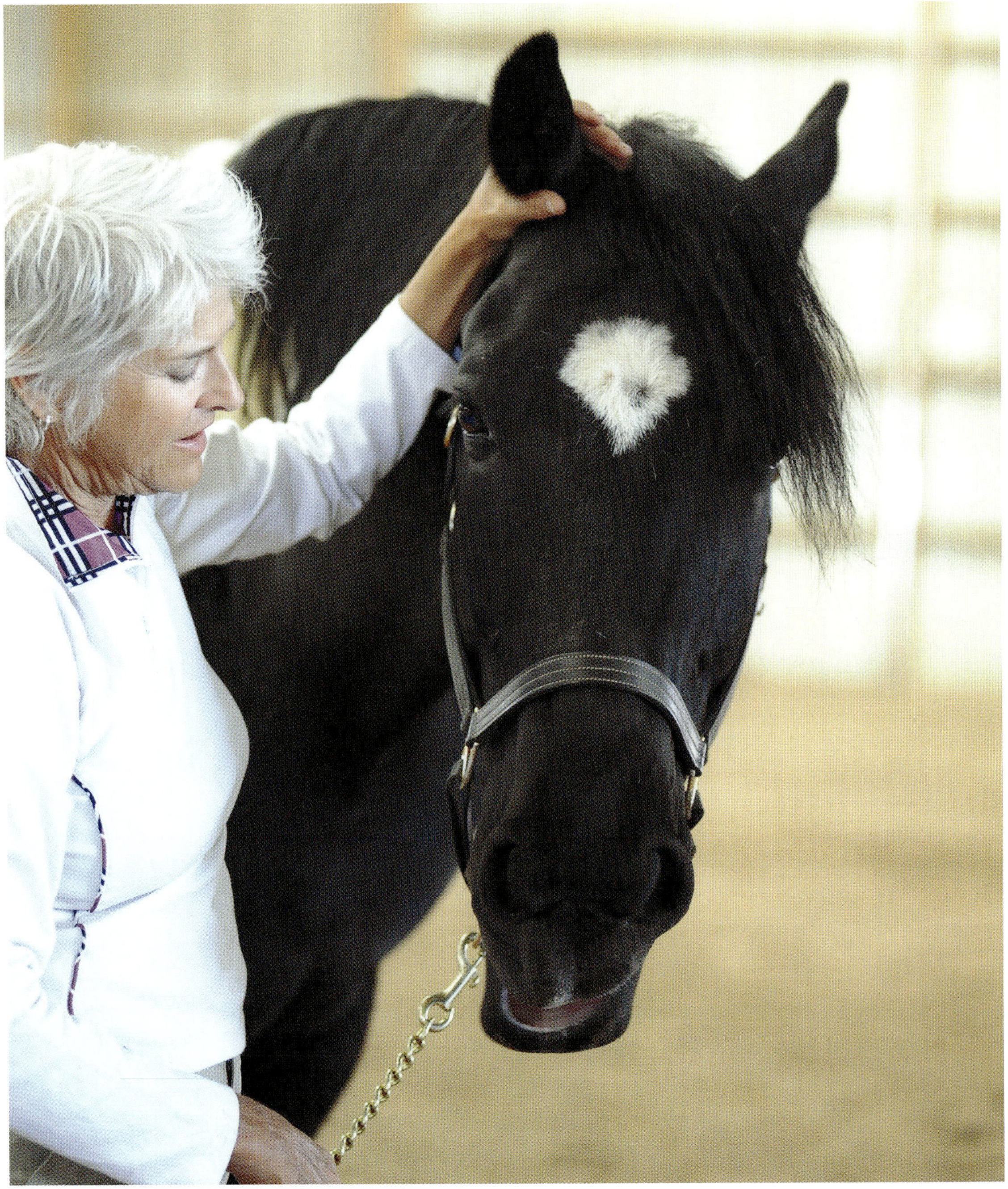

▶ **8.11** Beau enjoys a licking release as his ear changes create a better poll balance. He was longed often as a young horse and his head and poll imbalances are part of a front- and hind-end compensation pattern.

There are excellent sources of evaluation and discussion regarding hyperflexion in collected riding. I mention it briefly since it remains common in the horse world. The results of hyperflexion devastate the horse. It's important to recognize that it causes damage both emotionally and physically. Your responsibility for the horse's comfort and security is a foundation of riding. The riders who seek an advanced relationship with the horse have choices regarding their team's participation in riding, whether professional or amateur. We all acknowledge that our refusal to recognize the horse's limits can bring some very unwanted risks to riders, not to mention talented horses.

The physical growth of body consciousness is also a spiritual expansion for the horse. Like you, he has a choice to feel more or feel less. When the body's fascia flows well without compression, it brings "space" into compressed tissue. The space is felt as "light." This is why the consciousness increases when you feel more "in" your body. The increase in physical feeling and consciousness brings energy to meet life. Suddenly, more is possible on every level. The impossible healing has occurred in many cases. Things we thought the horse would be stuck with forever are gone, sometimes immediately.

There is always more space to find inside the horse and yourself. This expansion of consciousness initiates a new relationship with the horse and yourself based on the truth of how you both really feel. You find your true desire for relating to the horse, instead of taking your goals from an outside source. This truthful interaction with the horse, based on your true physical reality, brings peace and trust instead of pressure and fear.

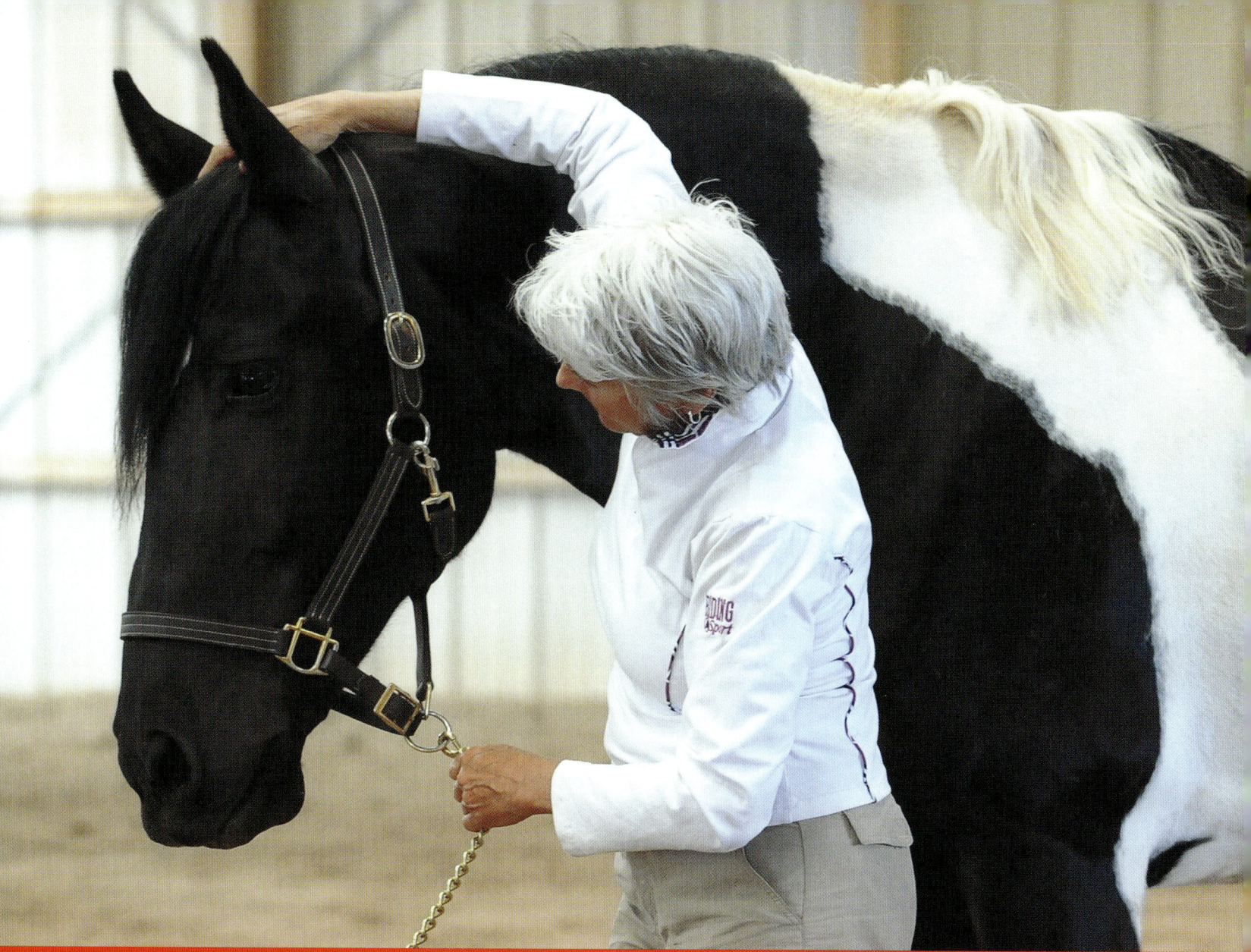

9 | Communicating with the Horse

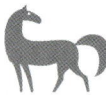

It's Not Just for Experts

Horse people all communicate with their horses. Some of us speak aloud to them while others don't. Here's an amazing fact: horses are telepathic. I learned this early on, in many sessions. The horses knew when I was afraid, upset, or nervous. I couldn't hide any feeling, especially a strongly emotional one, from horses. My feelings and inner comments were transferred to the horses, whether I liked it or not.

I was working at a barn one day where a trainer was hostile. The intelligent German horse I was working with commented, "You're nervous." I knew I couldn't lie to him. I replied with the mental message, "I'm upset at your trainer." I said what upset me. He accepted my reply. He didn't react with dominance, although he felt my imbalance. Our session went well.

This experience was a breakthrough for me. Suddenly, the complexities of my human world could be mentioned honestly, without fear. The horse may or may not reply, but he does listen. I suddenly realized that judging the horse and his condition was not only unprofessional to the horse, but it also blocked good work results. How can a horse feel a recovery when we are thinking about how terribly he moves, looks, or behaves? I saw that my attitude could block good relationships with horses. This new awareness of horse telepathy was a serious motivator for me to maintain an open, quiet mind when around them.

Some horse owners agree animal communication is possible and others do not feel such communication exists. Still others don't want to attempt direct dialogue at all, even if it's possible. There is room for every viewpoint. We all choose our comfort zone of intimacy with horses, just as we do with our human relationships. We don't need to feel guilty for not attempting constant intimacy. For many, the ideal is intimacy balanced with privacy, and comments are welcomed by both sides.

Telepathy with Horses

Telepathy is actually simply sending thoughts or pictures and receiving them. You can talk to your horse directly, both aloud and telepathically. When your behavior is honestly noted to the horse, you can explain when it is not about him. The lack of blame clears the air for both of you.

If you are nervous with your horse due to your own fears, you can tell him what's bothering you, or even that you need to learn more to be comfortable. He'll understand this. Incredibly, the horse knows that your emotions can rule his life. Even more incredibly, he doesn't resent you for this authority. He just wants to have a good day and feel secure. If your temper and irritations aren't about him, so much the better; you can tell him directly and remove the guesswork. The phrase, "I'm angry but it's not about you," offers great relief.

Here's a secret I discovered: if we have a quiet, blank mind, the horse shares his viewpoint as he chooses. This sharing often surfaces in the human mind like a

> "Horses force us to face our shadow selves. Once we do that, we discover much greater freedom, exhilaration and inspiration as we go forward in life."
>
> —*Chris Irwin, author of* Horses Don't Lie

thought or idea. It's a simple process. When our mind is busy and full of chattering thoughts or details of our human life, we'll miss these inputs. They are easy to miss because they are quiet, usually brief insights, and they slip, unnoticed, through your mind quickly. The comments slip in without quotation marks telling us that it's coming from the horse. Many times, we ignore the information and ideas that arrive this quietly. Often, we call them "insights." We're not sure where they came from, but they are helpful information.

Once we hear more than a few, if our minds are open, we notice that they have a characteristic tone and voice. We even notice a sense of humor. The remarks will offer tips or comments about situations. "She's my friend," or, "We don't get along." I have heard comments like, "The dog is gone." Or, as one horse commented, "At least she's honest," when a rider scolded her horses for continually grazing during a ride.

Go Ahead—Give It a Try

An easy way to practice telepathy is to start with a dog or cat. Here's how to begin: Look at the pet directly and ask a question mentally. A short, easy-to-answer question is best. "Do you like your food?" Or, if you have more than one pet, ask one if he likes the other, or how he feels about the other. The answers may surprise you. This is a great way to check on how the pet's life is going or if something is wrong.

After practice with a dog or cat, the horse is next. Again, ask easy questions with simple answers. No tricks here. If you don't believe in telepathy, you can ask skeptically. But then, you can't be surprised if the horse chooses not to answer. You can ask if he likes his

neighbor horse, or if he likes his food. Does the saddle fit? How does he feel? These are all useful questions to ask horses and open the channel for more intimacy, if you choose it.

Telepathy is very helpful to "clear the air" when we're upset or there's been events churning up the barn area. Again, the horse may not answer, but notice that he usually looks at you, in the eye, with understanding. Many horses and dogs make short comments or statements. "I'm a dog," replied the terrier when his owner angrily asked why he ran off in a parking lot. "Good to see you," said a horse when I returned to a barn not visited in many months. These are simple comments, but they show the open channel of communication.

An owner was frustrated when loading a horse to take him to an event. The horse, very happy at home, refused to load. The owner cajoled and tried treats, to no avail. Finally, the owner said, "We're going to see the children." She then loaded her other horse as a companion. The gelding looked at her and asked, "Is this a trick?" The owner laughed and said no. The horse looked at her suspiciously for a few moments, then loaded reluctantly. He was amazed when they did indeed visit a class of children who were thrilled to have horses come to their day camp.

There are many professional animal communicators offering a service that informs an owner of her horse's viewpoint and experiences. This service is very helpful for those who find themselves unable or unwilling to establish a direct communication with their horses. Professional animal communicators sometimes offer long discussions that they had with talkative horses. A stream of consciousness communication pattern brings that kind of information from a horse.

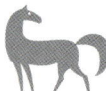

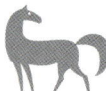

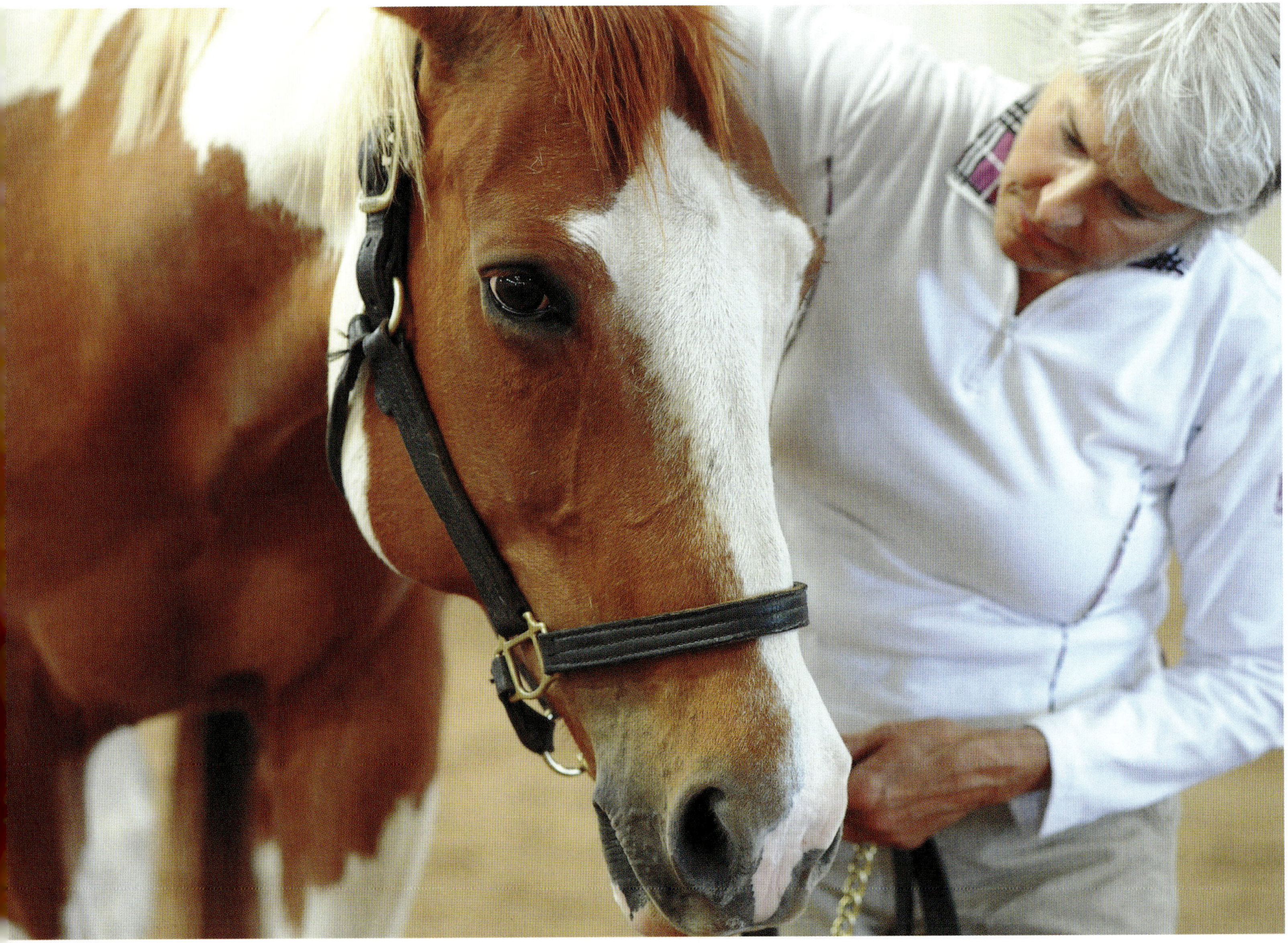

9.1 Scout's face shows conscious recognition of his change in his entire being. This conscious expression is a good example of the "light pipes" or fascia bringing consciousness into a dark, or compressed area. In these moments you need to have a clear and receptive mind, unclouded with thoughts that might interfere with fascia changes.

It is fascinating and often useful to hear the horse talk about situations or events in his life. The conversations tell you that the horse sees his environment very clearly. Like people, horses often choose their "sticking points," regarding conflict or choices and they tell you exactly what they see.

Each horse has his own particular character, just like we do. Some are interested in growth and others are more interested in being comfortable. Some horses like work, others like to relax in their paddocks. Some are open-minded, others not. Intelligence varies. Heart varies. Every horse has his own personality—some are cheerful, some are humorous, and some are skeptical. Others are "solid citizens" and some are mischievous.

Many owners tell me that their horses "picked them out" when they were looking for a horse. The story of looking for one kind of horse and bringing home a completely different one is common. What these stories share is that the horse selected that person to move himself into a new life. They look at us with a focused expression of connection and we are entranced by them. Then, the dance begins. A well-known example is the story of how Harry De Leyer, owner of the famous jumper Snowman (the "Eighty-Dollar Champion"), spoke of how the horse looked Harry in the eye from the truck bound for the slaughterhouse the night that Harry first encountered him.

Much good will is gained when we humans take the time to clear our minds and let the horse add his input. Not all riders want to factor in a horse's input; however, for those that do, there is a choice to listen. Here's an example: I bring out a saddle pad to tack up with and a thought suddenly comes in, "That saddle pad slips." Or, "I like that bit." At first, the insight seems to be my own.

As I developed a quieter mind, I heard the horse consistently. Preferences surfaced much more quickly, as I was willing to listen. Choices were simpler. There were no explanations, just the fact. I actually found this to be a great relief, especially regarding tack fitting well or a task being appropriate.

When I worried about particular horses getting along, they would tell me that they liked each other, despite the rough play—or, sometimes that they did not like each other and never would. I was then free to let a horse move on to a better fit. Like us, horses have chemistry with each other. When they aren't congruent, they will never get along well.

Recognition of the telepathic nature of horses helps us "know they know" what our loud, emotional thoughts are. We are not hiding anything from them with language, technical terms or false kindness. They know who we are. They know our intentions. This may terrify some riders and owners, but the truth is that many horses view their lives "professionally." They know they live at our pleasure and management. And, even if they don't agree with our decisions, horses do their best to get along with their circumstances.

Horses Share Their Stories

One day, before heading to the barn for work, I read a newspaper account of a barn fire in a distant state. The tragic, suspiciously started fire killed a family of horses, including a stallion, mares, and foals; the sad story upset me. As I drove to the barn, mental clearance of all thoughts was important. One session that morning was with a Friesian gelding. At the session end, he commented to me: "I know about the fire."

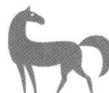

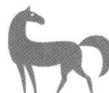

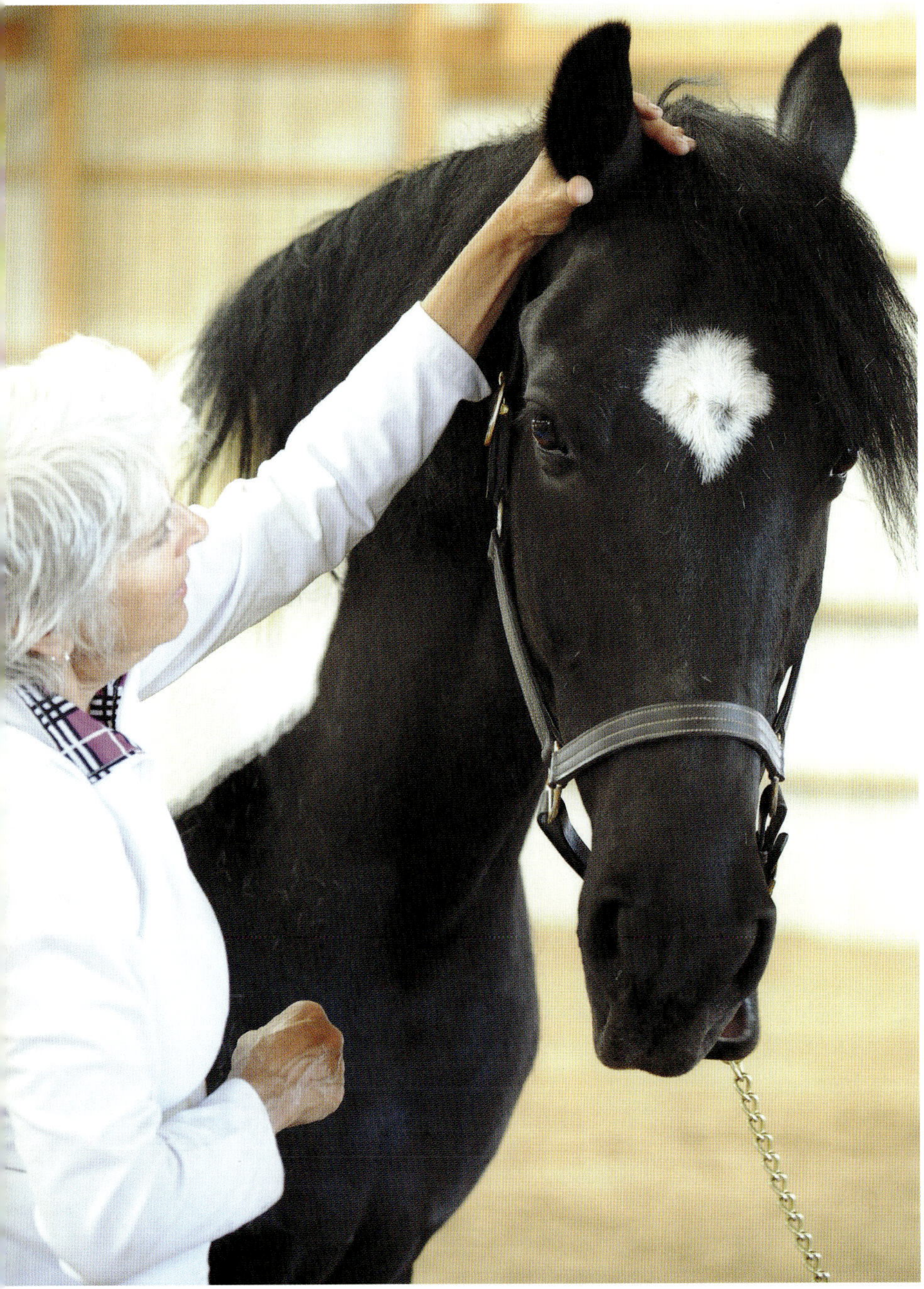

Tears came to my eyes. I was so astonished that I forgot to ask him how he knew. The answer came later from another horse. "We get the information." My understanding from this comment was that just as we use the internet to gain world news, the horse's telepathy brings him information, as well. He may not see the barn burning in Ohio, but he feels a terrible event and can sense that horses died. Horses may rely on telepathy, but they are not naïve. They know all about death, accidents, and other events. They don't hide from unpleasant truth. They accept these facts of life more completely than we humans do. This is another level of their service to us as friends in our lives.

A client shared an interesting story of horse communication. She was thinking about something regarding her horse while out in her pasture with him. A thought popped into her mind: "Shucks, I knew all about that." She told me with a laugh, "I would never use the word 'shucks,' so I knew it had to be him talking. It was so funny I laughed out loud." This same rider asked her horse how he liked his new paddock and barn after the family moved. "Everything's hunky-dory," her gaited, country-bred horse replied. She was delighted by his humor.

Another example is how a rider with a horse that expressed behavior problems suddenly experienced a headache. "I was thinking about him, and suddenly I felt a headache," she recalled. She mentioned this headache to her own therapist. "Well,

◄ **9.2** Beau responds with complete attention and cooperation to my wrapping his ear. My mind is open to receiving his thoughts and ideas.

he has a headache!" the therapist commented. The owner suddenly knew part of why the horse behaved so aggressively and she knew what her options were. He hurt and needed help.

Once, when working with an imported Warmblood, the horse offered a comment. "I'm not a dressage horse," he said. His back was hurting and collection was not easy for him. The horse knows how he can best be kept sound and use his abilities. He also knows what tasks he likes best. If he's continually put into work that is physically or temperamentally unsuitable, physical and emotional problems result, just as humans have problems when forced into jobs we can't do or don't like.

"I know about war," said a huge German Warmblood. "I've been in battle," he added. "It was my job and I didn't mind." He was a dressage horse, but the comment revealed the interconnectedness of time and life, although many people might find this impossible to believe.

An experienced Grand Prix dressage horse, Prince, was not behaving well. For over a week, his owner struggled with trying to ride in their usual way. The horse was erratic, fidgety, and wouldn't settle in for safe riding. He got particularly upset when being led or ridden near the travel trailer and the hay barn nearby. We attempted to communicate with Prince and he said, "Something is wrong—danger!"

What could it be? The large boarding facility was well maintained and managed. We imagined distant problems and complex issues as the danger source. But we soon found out what the danger was: a propane tank inside the travel trailer used as a residence for stable workers exploded. Prince, who lived in the barn nearby, broke out of his paddock and galloped away, inspiring

a few other terrified horses to bolt as well. The trailer was destroyed, but fortunately no one was inside at the time. Also, fortunately, the hay barn next door was safe.

We humans couldn't smell the propane leak or hear it, but Prince could, although he couldn't identify what he knew. The lesson here: When a horse is suddenly acting out, check and recheck possible problems. Simple questions can lead the horse to answers that we can understand. When a horse is uncharacteristically upset, there's a very good reason.

I've had horses send me pictures of an event that occurred to them. These are brief and not photographic images, but a soft, perhaps partial image of the

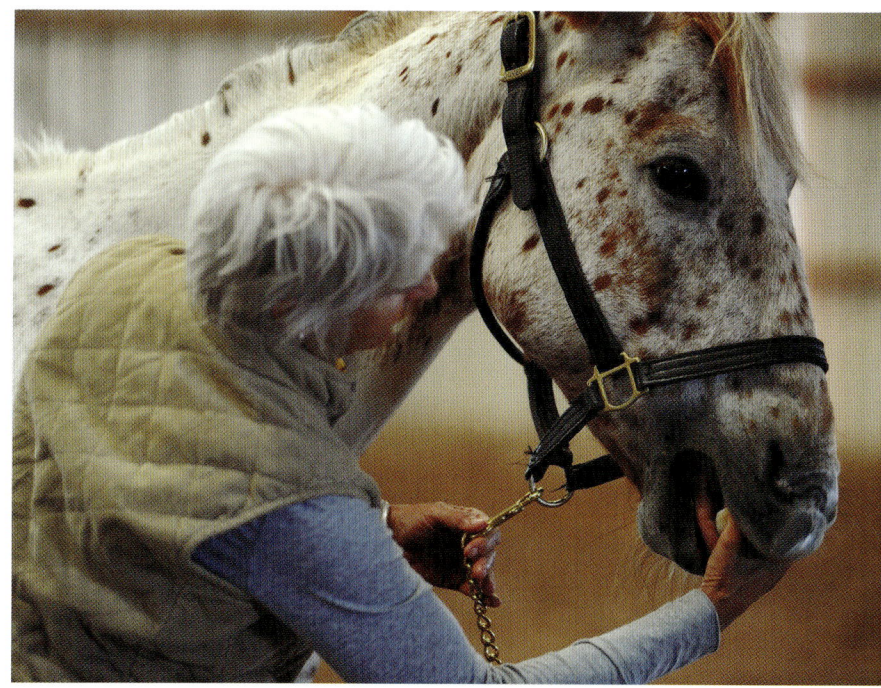

▲ **9.3** Remy ponders his fascia changes as he accepts a front lip release. Remy feels a new connection with himself and with me.

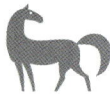

event or situation that caused them trouble. The picture often describes an accident, or perhaps an event, which occurred when the horse was under different ownership, or long ago in early life when no human was present. Some horses, however, will communicate little about even a difficult history. Like the person who has experienced a great amount of adversity or trauma but says little about it, some horses simply define their difficult past as "experience." I am always astonished by the generosity of horses and their acceptance of their reality.

Make Space for Hearing the Horse

Think about it, horses evolved with highly sensitive instincts to survive. As many notable trainers and equine practitioners have noted, horses have highly refined social structures and behavior codes. They are constantly assessing their environments for safety, comfort, and status. Why wouldn't the horse develop an ability to hear human decisions and thoughts, if they could? It is an evolutionary skill to adapt well to the human environment. Consequently, they have plenty of motivation to understand our human mind and cultivate adaptive advantages to get along more comfortably.

As we open ourselves to this kind of information and make space for hearing the horse, struggle melts away from the horse/human partnership. In case you wonder why you would want to spend the effort to pay attention, you might consider the comfort of being a real team instead of the panic and accidents that characterize many riding partnerships. In cases where the

Telepathic messages from the horse can arrive in pictures, too.

rider's goals don't align with the horse's actual ability, it's an opportunity to consider a new "dance partner."

Like human partnerships, horses want a happy, productive, and comfortable life with their owner, not stress and fear. The saying, "Nice people, bad marriage," applies to horse-and-rider partnerships too. Guilt is not an ingredient for a good relationship with horses. If the "chemistry" isn't bringing happiness, the rider can free the horse and herself for a more comfortable situation.

An Opportunity for Honesty

At this point, some of you may be thinking with horror, "Oh, no! My horse knows what I think." The truth is yes, he does know, especially when your thoughts have a lot of emotion wrapped around them. Emotion is like a megaphone: horses are so highly tuned that the more emotional energy mixed in with your thoughts, the better they hear them!

This telepathic quality of being is one of the gifts of therapeutic horses. The horses used in therapy with humans have agreed to this service and nurture their human friends without fail. Like people, these horses are suited to relationship work: with autistic children, veterans, and other trauma cases. They intimately serve their clients with pleasure.

Some riders might feel that direct communication with horses, or attempting such communication, creates stress for them. Again, you can choose your level of intimacy with horses. However, the fact is, the human-created environment for horses is so full of controls and stress anyway that the horses may experience

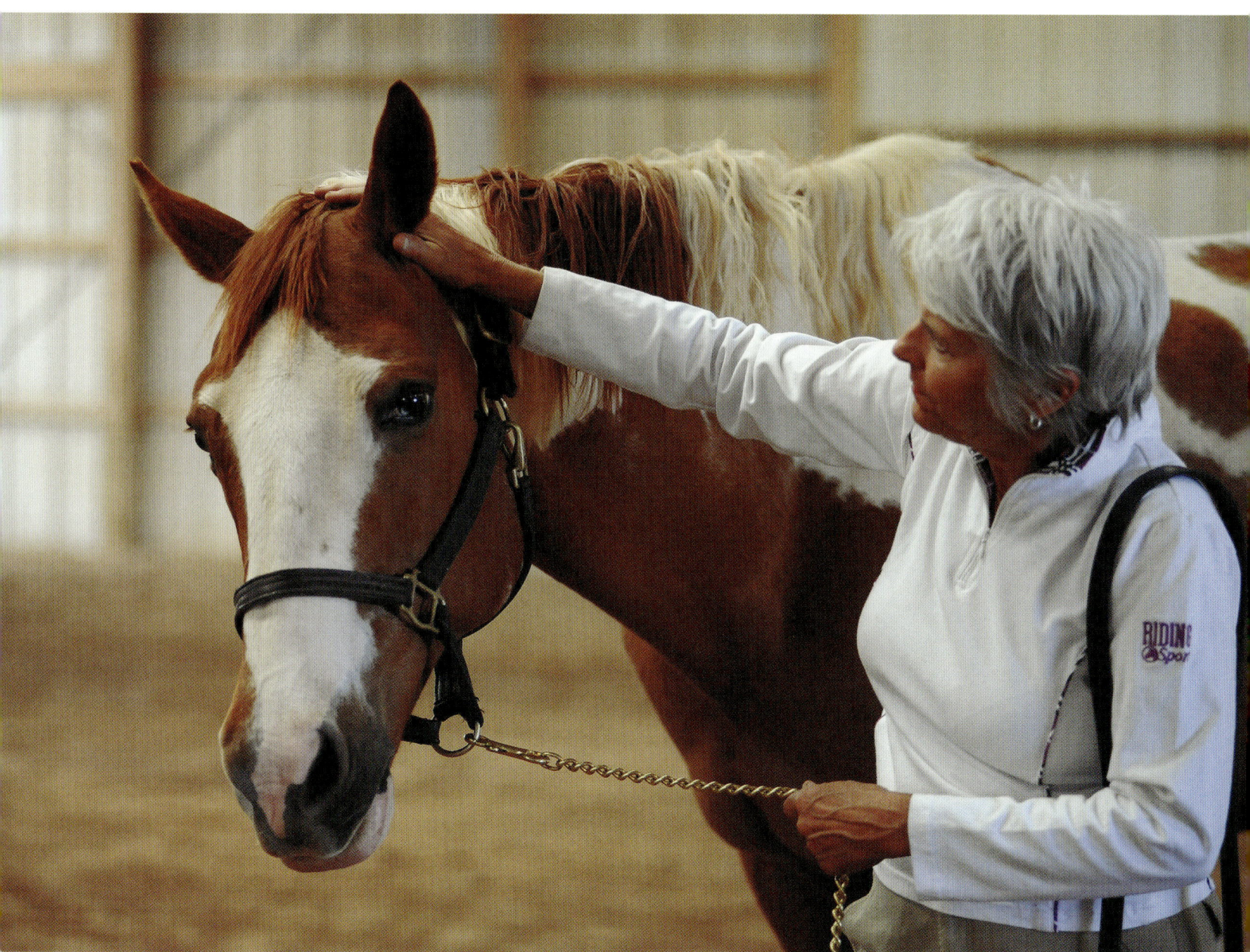

▲ **9.4** Scout shows the conscious change of a Still Point. This consciousness is a bridge between the horse and rider and is the gift of partnership.

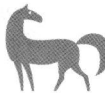

a huge responsibility just being with you, and partnering in your riding goals.

You can choose to develop more personal responsibility in this partnership, or not, as your case may be. A magical, inspired partnership is a vital ingredient to all the champion performances in the horse world, as well as in many human sports and endeavors.

Yet, for those who are not interested in such intimacy, both sides of the relationship can decide to limit the communication channels, just as people do in their human relationships. There are many horses that are excellent mounts for their riders and yet live a rather aloof life. These horses don't nicker at the stall door when you come, or stand watching you clean tack. They drift off to their own corner for quiet time. They are often easy to handle and have a good work ethic, but they prefer a private existence of their own. Many human and equine partnerships are strictly business affairs, and this often succeeds well for the pair. That's a choice, too.

Many horses consider themselves professionals. They show up for their job, but they also don't take us personally. This is a great advantage, as you know from your own work-related relationships. This choice relieves the human from caretaking for the horse's experience, if that is not his choice. Sometimes, if your life is particularly busy and demanding, you can offer the comment to your horse, "I have human problems to work on."

An ability to be present for input is a powerful tool for us, rather than filling our minds with self-blame or guilt over situations that brought problems. For those who resist or dislike the concept of telepathy, another approach might be to call this communication "conscious empathy" with the horse. Any channel that allows you to creatively accept inspiring input is worth considering. In my experience, the horse is often waiting to connect with you. After all, his own happiness and survival depends on his relationship with you. A desire for true partnership, with mutual trust, respect, and affection motivate you in your interactions with the horse. There is no better goal.

"I want to be a lead mare," said a young horse, behaving very ambitiously in her herd, bossing the other older horses about the paddock. This character showed as a yearling. As many trainers and horse people know, character does not change. Just as people are born with a character and personality, so are horses. This is another reason why if the chemistry fit isn't good, it's a kindness to let the horse move on to a more suitable situation. Often, we hear the debate of keeping or selling the horse. The horse knows all about this. You can save time and worry by checking in with him on how his life feels to him and if his work suits him. You can even comment to him why a new home may be needed. You'll be surprised at how practical horses are!

Horses also often know when their time to pass from life on earth has come. I've heard them say, "I don't know if I can make it." Or even, "I don't want to live now that my friend is gone." As with human relationships, we can choose to express our love for them or decide to be reserved. Horses do not blame us either way.

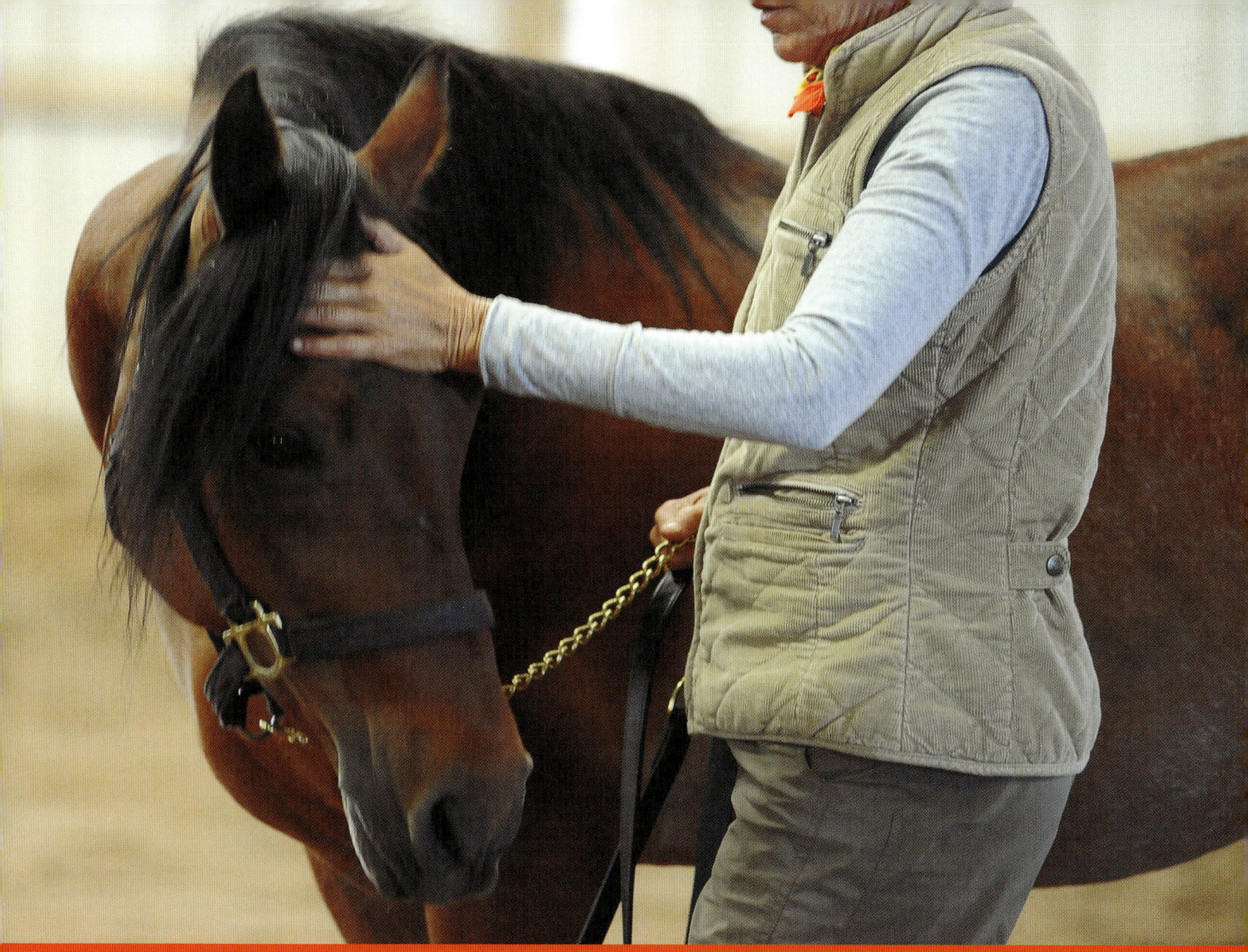

10 | Staying with the Miracle

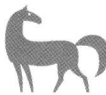

Like Any Dance Pair

When you look around, you see many new modalities available now for horses to progress. With a new awareness of the important role of fascia, the choices simplify. With this work, your horse becomes much more fit. And if you use my suggestions about developing the walk, halts, and shoulder-in, you'll find your own skills greatly improve, as well. Your own fitness in riding will increase, along with your horse's condition.

The other side of the fit horse is being able to ride him. Like any dance pair, balance is required by both partners, not just the lead dancer. The horse cannot always correct the rider's "stuff." Riders are wise to be evaluated and have regular fascia-change work themselves. A body professional, friend, or riding coach can help you check your alignment. Mirrors show you how you stand. Look for enlargements or smaller parts on yourself, as you do with the horse. An injury or broken limb will bring asymmetry along with compensations. Replacement parts can also affect how balanced you are and they should be included in this assessment.

The Body Map

I include the body map as a useful tool to organize notes for your sessions with the horse (fig. 10.1). When you keep notes of where you start, it reminds you later about how much changed. Remember, an amazing aspect of fascial transformation is that as you progress away from trauma memory with Soma-Emotional Recall, the old problem fades away emotionally. You then forget that there was a major issue at all. The old tying or loading struggles grow faint and you recall them almost like

an old photo: you think it wasn't such a big deal after all, despite the fact it may have been a pretty big deal for you or the horse more than once.

Truthful records remind you what it was like, how the fascia changes brought solutions, and what your horse is like today. This brings gratitude and acceptance for you both. Human gratitude and appreciation is an oasis of security and peace for the horse.

The body map is easy to use for notes and recording limitation areas, stiffness, and gait problems. As your sensitivity improves, you may need less record keeping, but it is a powerful tool at the start, and especially with a horse enmeshed in major difficulties and imbalances. For professionals, the body map also helps set training or work tasks more honestly, with the horse's skills and limitations in mind. You cannot train for collection, in fairness, when a horse has imbalanced hindquarters or tight shoulders.

Balanced Impulsion

Impulsion is another new trait the fit horse reveals. As your horse balances, he'll move forward with energy. This can feel like an out-of-control horse to a rider used to a sluggish, imbalanced horse with little power. Experienced riders say that riding a collected horse with impulsion feels like a surging of continual power as the back lifts, almost like the horse will buck. As your horse improves, you must be ready.

Here's where the walk helps you become comfortable with the horse's new impulsion. In chapter 7, I discussed the importance of the walk in conditioning horses (see p. 115). Now that the horse is in condition, you still use the walk for maintenance. Walks

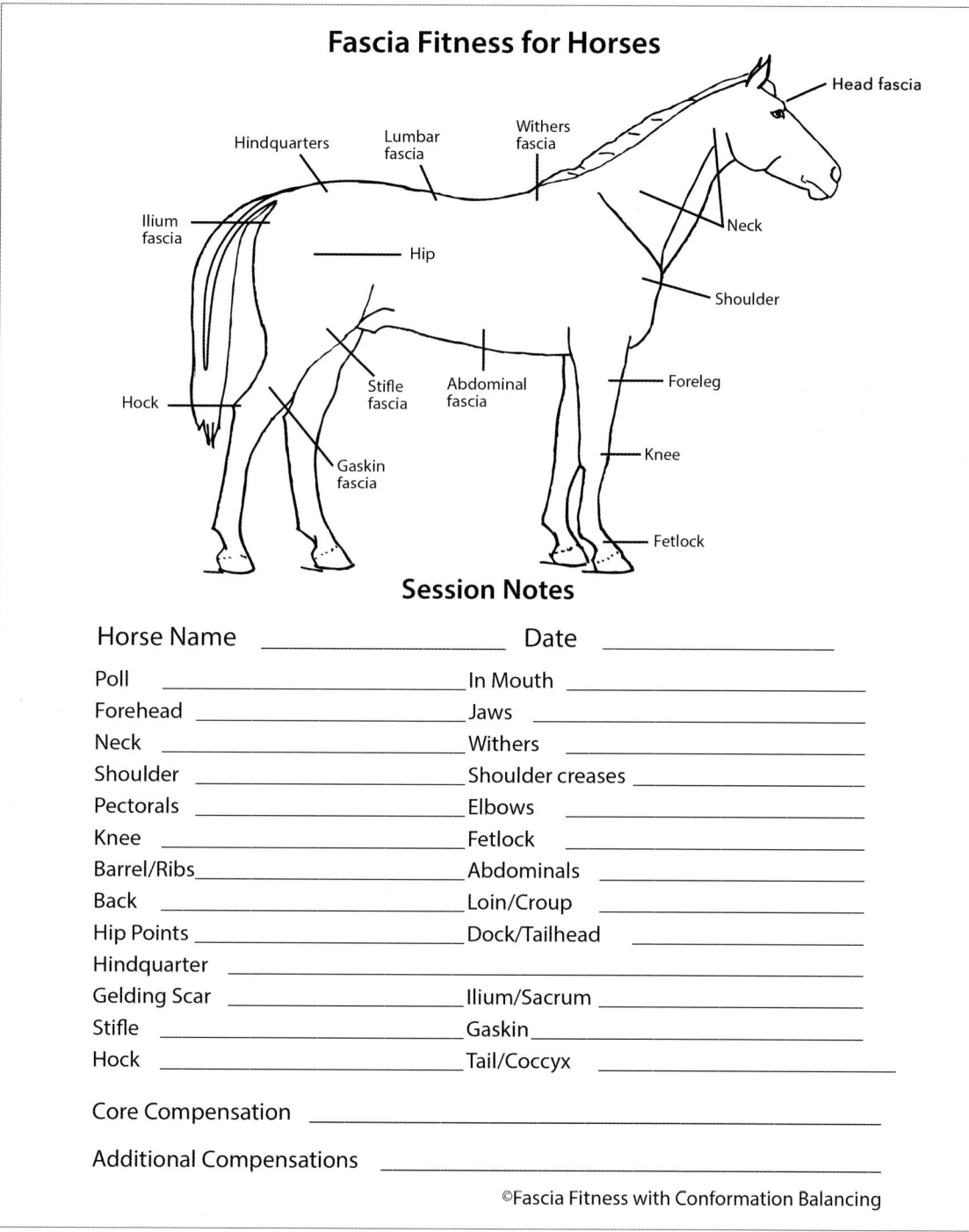

Fascia Fitness for Horses

Head fascia

Withers fascia

Lumbar fascia

Hindquarters

Neck

Ilium fascia

Hip

Shoulder

Stifle fascia

Abdominal fascia

Foreleg

Hock

Gaskin fascia

Knee

Fetlock

Session Notes

Horse Name _____ Date _____

Poll _____ In Mouth _____

Forehead _____ Jaws _____

Neck _____ Withers _____

Shoulder _____ Shoulder creases _____

Pectorals _____ Elbows _____

Knee _____ Fetlock _____

Barrel/Ribs_____ Abdominals _____

Back _____ Loin/Croup _____

Hip Points _____ Dock/Tailhead _____

Hindquarter _____

Gelding Scar _____ Ilium/Sacrum _____

Stifle _____ Gaskin_____

Hock _____ Tail/Coccyx _____

Core Compensation _____

Additional Compensations _____

©Fascia Fitness with Conformation Balancing

10.1 The body map with its basic checklist is a tool for recording the horse's progress. Be sure to date it by month and year.

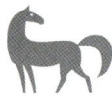

come at varied speeds (and that doesn't even begin to account for what is possible for gaited horses). The walk becomes a "regular routine" during rides. New ability shows in the walk, as does a relapse of any kind. But impulsion prevents the walk from feeling tedious or slow.

Many riding books, trainers, and workshops teach that the greatest sin in equitation is pulling back on the reins. As I discussed earlier, this "braking" of the horse with the reins damages the horse's back and hindquarters, making collection painful, not to mention creating strain in his neck, poll, and jaw. A fit horse consciously feeling his body tissue is less agreeable to being forced into damaging positions. This brings you full circle to why fitness is a process, not a final goal.

A New Relationship with the Horse

Conformation Balancing brings a new consciousness to riding, which expands your relationship with the horse into new confidence for both parties. This transformation brings a huge new energy of a different kind into your relationship (fig. 10.2). When you ride, you'll notice your horse's responsiveness in a new way. Instead of thinking, "He won't," you begin to think, "Maybe, he can't." The horse feels the shift, too. As he improves, you're pleased and you enjoy his advances. The horse notices that enjoyment also. Life improves for him as he does more good things than bad. Grooming becomes more than brushing off dirt or preparing for a ride.

Watching the horse move now has a whole new purpose as you see the amazingly subtle, yet important

> As fascia limits are relieved, the comfortable horse relaxes into mental poise and physical balance.

progress of the horse's fascia changes and new freedom of movement. Your new appreciation for the horse inspires the horse, too. He becomes aware of himself in an expansive way, instead of attempting to meet a constant chattering checklist of behavior patterns that dull his senses and yours. As body competency increases, freshness occurs routinely as both partners explore the new possibilities.

The difference between humans and horses is profound. Humans often use mental approaches to resolve problems. Horses live in their body's experience of the situation. Training is a layer of civilization, but it won't override what is held inside the horse's body.

Intuition is helpful as you explore the horse's body. Curiosity helps you find limits and compensations, and your experience grows. Practice is how your skill increases to help advance your horse's fitness. The feeling of being helpless regarding injury in the horse will leave you as you understand the horse's "internet" better.

Your own confidence inspires trust in the horse regarding your leadership. He knows you will take care of him because you have already improved his quality of life. He feels better every time you work with him. Best of all, when you come to the horse, it's not about your own goals, but you now offer him ways to be more comfortable in his own skin. With practice, your hands find a myriad of fascial sensations.

Stiff sheets of adhesions, worm-like strings and cords, thin wiry twinges, waves of heat release are a few of the sensations you learn to recognize immediately with your hands. Again, it's not about identifying

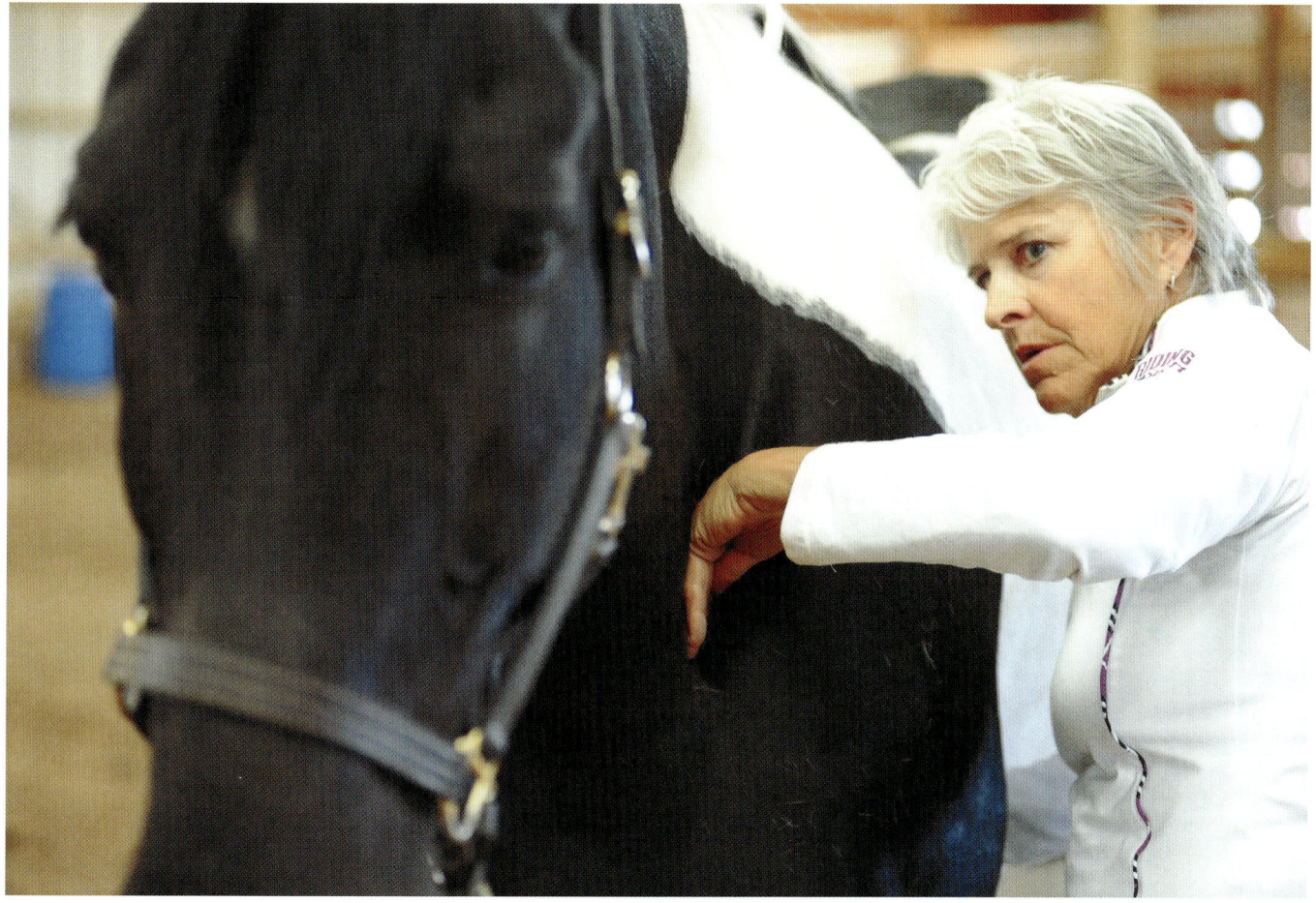

▲ **10.2** Beau shows intelligence as he focuses on his shoulder fascia change. A Still Point is where the most change happens for the horse. When I help him find it, a door opens in our relationship.

carefully exactly what they are, it's about letting yourself develop a kinesthetic intelligence that can guide your connection with the tissue.

As I said back in the beginning of the book, computer work isn't learned in two hours or even two weeks. The Conformation Balancing process, like computer work, relies on developing layers of understanding and increasing sensitivity to the operating systems. The fascia-change process is about where the changes happen and how they might connect with the rest of the horse's body and movement. You learn to look far away from the source of stiffness itself—diagonally, laterally,

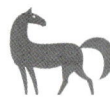

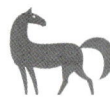

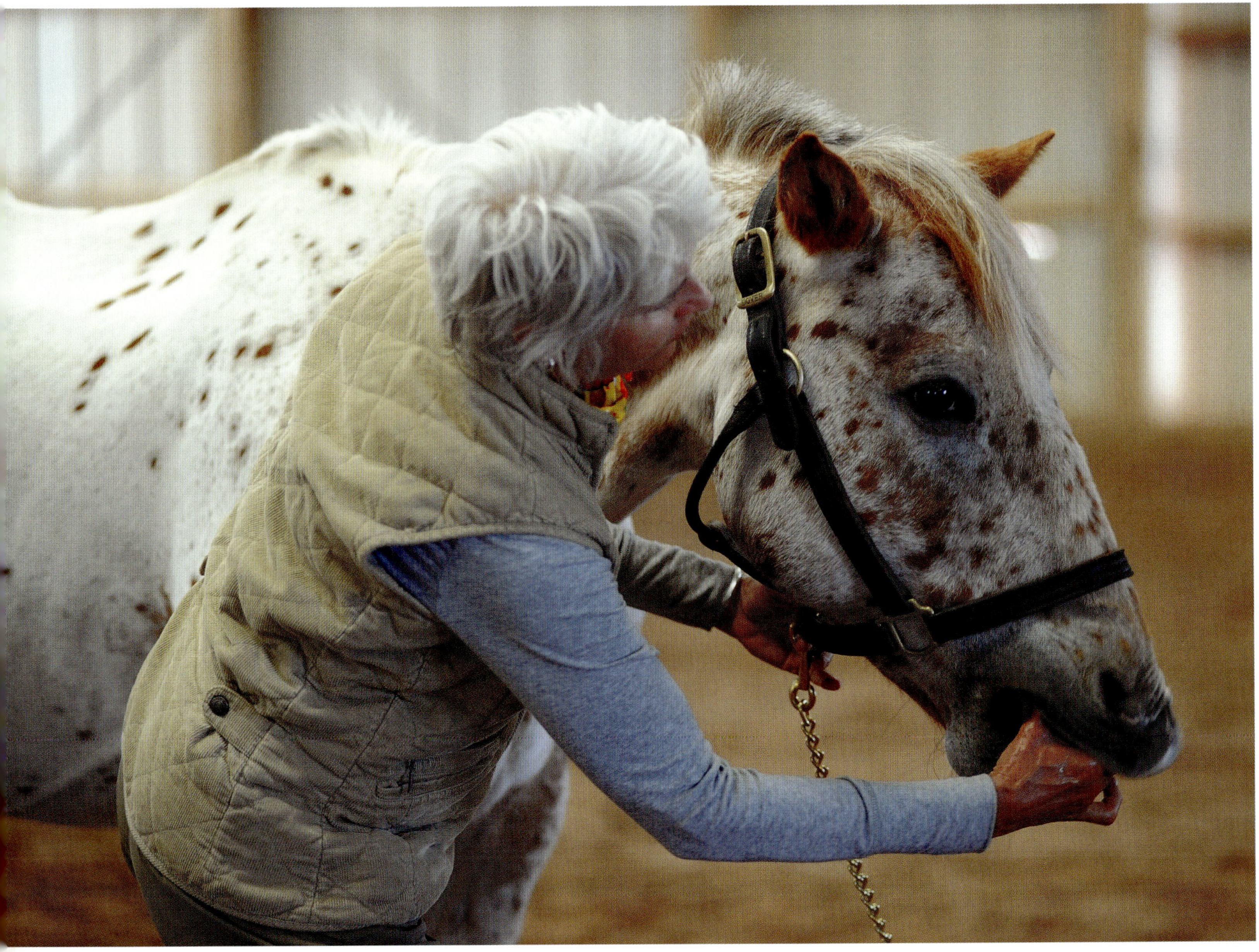

▲ **10.3** Remy pushes into his head balancing with this front lip change. This is a high strain area for horses and progress here transforms an anxious horse into a poised one.

or wherever you may find it. Poll imbalance controls the hindquarters development, as you know now. This book offers all the basic tools for this new journey with the horse.

How to Fit It In

Now that you have these new tools for helping your horse, there's another question. How do you fit this bodywork into your barn time? As I've said in nearly every chapter, you use the time available. Short sessions are as effective as long ones; a lot of change is accomplished in 15 minutes on a regular basis. Or a half-hour, twice a week, might suit you better. Younger horses prefer short sessions. Older, stiff horses savor repeated hour sessions. However you work it, an advance in any body "site" spreads its message to all parts of the horse. As you've seen, changes in the tail resonate in the head.

The paradox of fascia is that its very complexity allows simple change for lasting resolution. A little work goes a long way, with consistent practice. All you need to do is offer warm hands to balance tight areas of the fascia

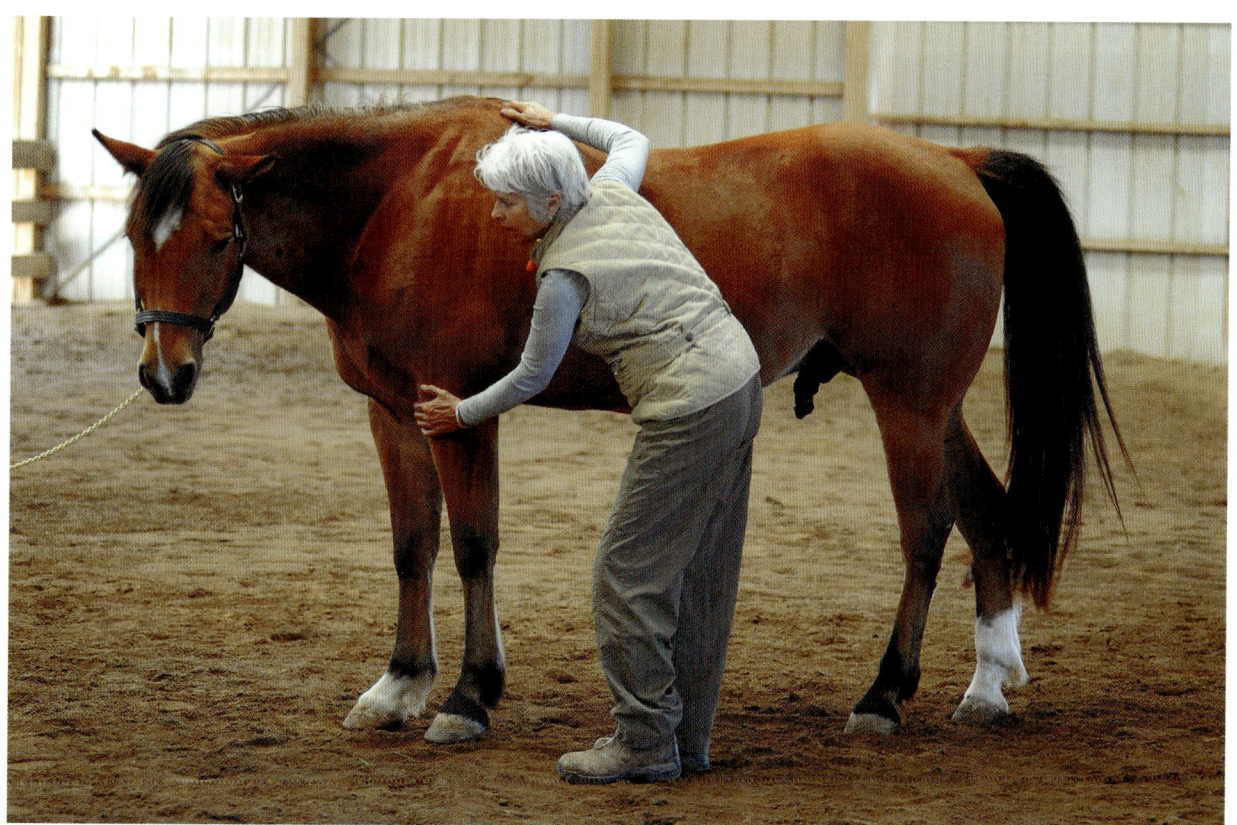

◀ **10.4** EZ shows receptivity to the bodywork partnership well here. Notice his plumed tail, curving neck, and natural head carriage. The fascia is a miraculous, self-intelligent path to help the horse make progress. Short or long sessions work well; any session length is better than none.

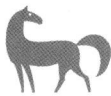

whenever you feel like it. You offer change often when there are limits. You also offer change to prevent limits and maintain full range of motion.

It's an important fact that this fascia-change work saves you riding struggles. Regardless of how you fit Conformation Balancing into your horse time, it always helps your horse progress. There is no lost time, no matter how little seems to be happening. Unlike rides where you both return to the barn annoyed with each other, fascial changes always bring advances. Many of the tasks that relied on repetitive behavior are completed very quickly and well, once the horse is balancing. That ease of movement in your horse brings the motivation for the work. The rewards are huge.

This astonishing process of change and balancing is lasting and progressive. As you learn to recognize the horse's change, you help the horse and yourself, too. You become more and more sensitive to movement and quality of competency. This new consciousness for the horse's movement brings you new insights into how you can partner with the horse. Truly, the horse's progressive consciousness through a smoothly flowing internet of fascia brings you into a new dimension of partnership with your horse.

Recommended Resources

Architecture of Human Living Fascia: Cells and Extracellular Matrix as Revealed by Endoscopy by Jean-Claude Guimberteau and Colin Armstrong (Handspring Publishing, 2015)

Craniosacral Therapy by John Upledger and J. D. Vredevoogd (Eastland Press, 1983)

Dancing with Horses by Klaus Ferdinand Hempfling (Trafalgar Square Books, 2012)

Fascial Dysfunction: Manual Therapy Approaches edited by Leon Chaitow (Handspring Publishing, 2014)

The Field by Lynne McTaggart (Harper Perennial, 2008)

The Heart of Listening: A Visionary Approach to Craniosacral Work by Hugh Milne (North Atlantic Books, 1998)

Myofascial Release by John Barnes (Rehabilitation Services, Inc., 1990)

Physical Therapy and Massage for the Horse by Jean-Marie Denoix & Jean-Pierre Pailloux (Trafalgar Square Books, 2001)

Release The Potential: A Practical Guide to Myofascial Release for Horse & Rider by Doris Halstead and Carrie Cameron (Half Halt Press, 2000)

Touching Light: How to Free Your Fiber-Optic Fascia by Ronelle Wood (CreateSpace, 2015)

Tug of War: Classical Versus "Modern" Dressage by Dr. Gerd Heuschmann (Trafalgar Square Books, 2007)

Index

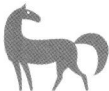

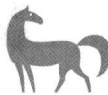